ETHICAL ISSUES IN
HOME HEALTH CARE

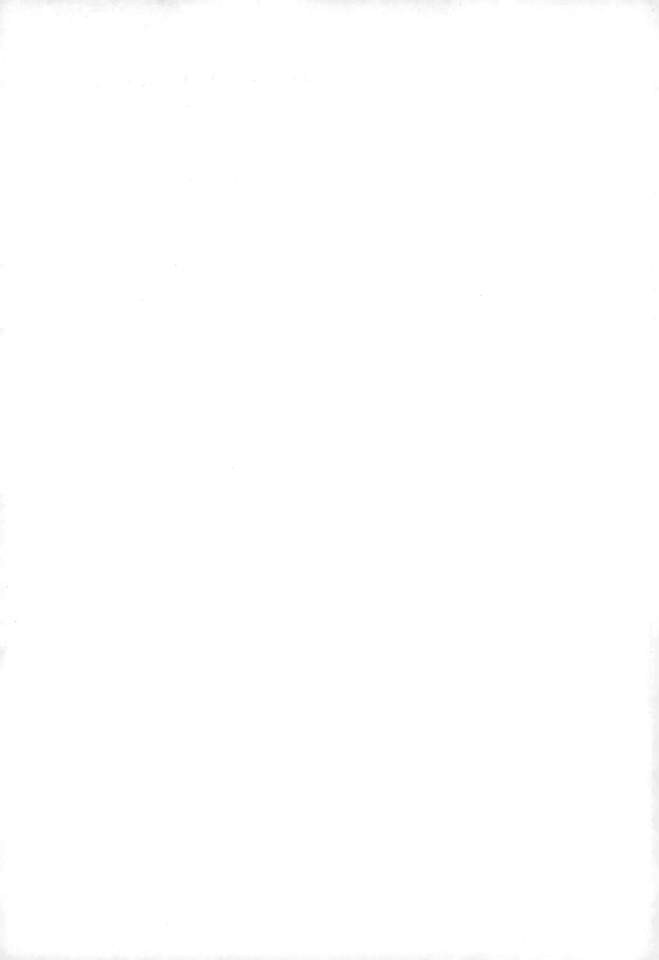

Second Edition

ETHICAL ISSUES IN HOME HEALTH CARE

By

SHERI SMITH, Ph.D.

Rhode Island College
Providence, Rhode Island

ROSALIND EKMAN LADD, Ph.D.

Wheaton College
Norton, Massachusetts

LYNN PASQUERELLA, Ph.D.

University of Rhode Island
Kingston, Rhode Island

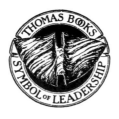

CHARLES C THOMAS • PUBLISHER, LTD.
Springfield • Illinois • U.S.A.

Published and Distributed Throughout the World by

CHARLES C THOMAS • PUBLISHER, LTD.
2600 South First Street
Springfield, Illinois 62704

©2008 by CHARLES C THOMAS • PUBLISHER, LTD.

ISBN 978-0-398-07808-9 (hard)
ISBN 978-0-398-07809-6 (paper)

Library of Congress Catalog Card Number: 2008004196

With THOMAS BOOKS *careful attention is given to all details of man-
ufacturing and design. It is the Publisher's desire to present books that are satisfactory as to their physical qualities and artistic possibilities and appropriate for their particular use.* THOMAS BOOKS *will be true to those laws
of quality that assure a good name and good will.*

*Printed in the United States of America
CR-R-3*

Library of Congress Cataloging-in-Publication Data

Smith, Sheri, Ph.D.
  Ethical issues in home health care / by Sheri Smith, Rosalind Ekman
Ladd, Lynn Pasquerella. -- 2nd ed.
    p. cm.
  Ladd's name appears first on the earlier ed.
  Includes bibliographical references and index.
  ISBN 978-0-398-07808-9 (hard) -- ISBN 978-0-398-07809-6 (pbk.)
  1. Home care services--Moral and ethical aspects. 2. Home nursing--
Moral and ethical aspects. I. Ladd, Rosalind Ekman. II. Pasquerella,
Lynn. III. Title.
  [DNLM: 1. Home Care Services--ethics. 2. Ethics, Nursing. 3. Nurse-
Patient Relations--ethics.
WY 115 S659e 2008]

RA645.3.L33 2008
174.2--dc22

                                                                2008004196

For the many nurses who generously shared their stories with us.
R.E.L. and S.L.S.

For my uncle, Olney Fortier, in gratitude of his continous support and
deep and abiding commitment to intellectual pursuits.
L.P.

PREFACE

This book lets us listen to the voices of home health care nurses as they pose the ethical questions they encounter in their work. The cases presented in each chapter are fictionalized situations based on interviews conducted with home health care nurses in both hospital–sponsored and private agencies, in hospices, and in urban and rural settings. We have attempted to avoid the use of gendered pronouns, except in the discussion of cases, where their use reflects the fact that the majority of nurses in home health care are women.

Home health care is an increasingly important venue for nursing as advances in medical technology and cost-containing measures shift the ill population from hospital to home. The decrease in the length of hospital stays, with patients being discharged sooner and requiring more complex care, together with the aging of the population, has resulted in an increasing number of older, sicker, frailer patients being cared for at home. The rise of specialties such as geriatric case managers has also contributed to the possibility of more individuals being able to access services at home. As a consequence of these changes, home health care nurses may face a growing number of ethical questions and more complex ethical issues.

Not surprisingly, practicing nursing in the patient's home raises different kinds of ethical questions than are raised in hospital nursing. The general nursing literature addresses ethical issues, but little attention has been paid to the special circumstances of home health care and the fact that this kind of nursing requires different strategies for effective ethical responses.

Each chapter of the book is devoted to one of the main areas of concern for home health care nurses. Focusing on specific cases, it offers analysis and discussion of the ethical issues, cites legal requirements where relevant, and summarizes ethical criteria and practical strategies. Whether student or seasoned professional, the reader is afforded the opportunity to gain increased sensitivity to what counts as an ethical question and a better understanding of the critical thinking process that leads to careful, reasoned decisions about what to do. At the same time, reflection on the issues and attention to the reasoning process can aid in communicating with patients and families about the often emotion-laden decisions that constitute the core of home health care ethics.

In this second edition, the text has been revised to reflect new developments in nursing ethics. The discussion of confidentiality and privacy incorporates the requirements for safeguarding confidentiality of medical records and patient information created by the Health Insurance Portability and Accountability Act. The ethical requirements for culturally competent nursing care have been addressed in the chapter on respecting cultural differences. There is also an updated discussion of the provisions of the revised American Nurses Association Code of Ethics, including the Bill of Rights for Registered Nurses. In addition, some cases have been rewritten to accord with changes in medical technology and the term "patients" has been substituted for the earlier references to "clients."

New material has been added in the form of two additional Appendices. One appendix includes ten new cases which may be used for discussion in groups or for individual practice in ethical analysis. The second appendix discusses how to develop and use Ethics Committees within home health care agencies. There are also a number of new cases introduced within the various chapters.

There is one change in organization. The cases which introduce the topic of each chapter are discussed and analyzed as the last section in each chapter rather than being analyzed in a separate chapter at the end of the book.

ACKNOWLEDGMENTS

We are indebted to many individuals who both enriched our work and made it possible, beginning with the nurses who shared their stories with us and the agencies that provided us with access. Special recognition should be given to the Rhode Island State Nurses Association and to the nursing faculties at Rhode Island College and the University of Rhode Island. Several nursing scholars made unique contributions. From the project's inception, Mary E. Byrd's inspiration and advice have proven instrumental in the design and evolution of our research and the development of this book. Joanne Costello, Ph.D., A.P.R.N.-B.C., and Jane Williams, Ph.D., R.N., have also contributed enormously by offering insights into the nature of nursing practice in the home health care context. We are also grateful to Trudy C. Mulvey, M.S.N., R.N., C.S., and Maureen Newman, Ph.D., A.P.R.N., for their insights about home health care nursing. Professor Byrd, Ph.D., R.N., Professor Costello, and Professor Williams, together with Carol Reagan Shelton, Ph.D., R.N., and Patricia A. Thomas, Ph.D., R.N., assisted us by reading and commenting on drafts of chapters. Their efforts improved the book considerably, though any mistakes are, of course, our own. In addition, members of the planning committee, Virginia Tougas Conway, R.N., B.S., Mary Ellen M. Januario, R.N., Pamela L. McCue, M.S.N., R.N., and participants at the home health care conference "How Far Should We Go? Practical Approaches to Ethical Dilemmas: Managed Care, Noncompliance and End-of-Life Decisions" provided valuable feedback on many of the case studies we developed.

We also appreciate the support of friends, colleagues, and family members, whose encouragement was indispensable to us during the process of research and writing. We hope they know the extent of our gratitude.

Finally, we want to thank Beatrice M. Price for her excellent skills as an administrative assistant, which contributed to producing this manuscript.

CONTENTS

ETHICAL ISSUES IN
HOME HEALTH CARE

Chapter 1

ETHICAL DECISION MAKING

Ethical issues arise in home health care, as in human lives generally, in many diverse types of situations. Sometimes an issue arises because there is an important disagreement with others about what is right to do—a conflict that may have its origin in disagreement about fundamental moral values and principles. Perhaps the most confounding and most common issues, though, involve situations where it is initially unclear what is right, and individuals must resolve their own moral uncertainty in order to reach a decision. In all of these instances, ethical decision-making must have its foundation in a basic understanding of the nature of ethics and traditional moral ideas concerning right and wrong. Case 1 provides an example of a situation in home health care that raises a concern about what to do.

Case 1

I have a patient with cancer who is dying at home. Her two sisters are staying with her to take care of her. Because she is on morphine, she has experienced constipation, recently developed a partial bowel obstruction, and needs a colostomy. Last week she told me she didn't want the surgery because she didn't think her sisters could deal with it. As her condition has worsened, her sisters have noticed she is bloated and nauseated. They are pressuring me to tell them what is happening. **Should I support her decision to spare her family?**

General Issues

- **What is ethics?**
- **How should claims about rights be used in making ethical decisions?**

- **What role should consequences have in ethical decision-making?**
- **What other factors should be considered?**

INTRODUCTION

In Case 1, the nurse faces a classic ethical dilemma, that is, a conflict between two moral ideals. One ideal holds that nurses should respect a patient's right to make decisions, but here that ideal conflicts with the responsibility nurses also have to promote a patient's health and well-being. The decision the nurse must make in this situation is different from the clinical decisions she confronts every day, for this involves the kind of question that goes beyond facts. The uncertainty about what it is right to do cannot be resolved by gathering more factual information or even through further assessment of a patient's clinical condition. Instead, answering ethical questions requires skill in identifying the significant moral factors in a situation and then reasoning to a conclusion about the best course of action.

This case illustrates three important features of the special challenges home health care nurses face when ethical conflicts arise: First, although they are part of an interdisciplinary team, home health care nurses are usually the only professionals in the home when a decision must be made. Second, the home setting itself may be the source of moral concerns, for example, if obstacles exist that prevent ideal nursing interventions on behalf of a patient. Third, though their primary responsibility is to care for patients, nurses must also respond to concerns about family members or others who are caregivers. As a result, the ethical dilemmas nurses face in home health care are not only complex but also in some instances unique to the home setting.

Ideally, home health care nurses will be adept at thinking through solutions to ethical problems, without the benefit of immediate advice from professional colleagues, and they will be able to assist patients and families in understanding and coping with difficult decisions. These skills can be developed through thoughtful reflection on ethics and practice in ethical decision-making.

WHAT IS ETHICS?

Ethics involves critical reflection on fundamental moral beliefs, that is, beliefs about how to live, what has meaning and value, and which actions are morally right. The ultimate goal of careful reflection on these issues is a decision or a claim about morality that is thoughtful and well supported by reasons. Thus, reasonable answers to moral questions and good ethical decisions will be the result of critical thinking.

Laws and nursing codes of ethics offer legal standards and moral ideals for the practice of nursing, but they cannot substitute for ongoing critical thinking about ethical issues. Laws, for example, are not very helpful in determining what is ethically right to do, because they state legal standards that are often vague and which need to be interpreted. Because legal standards are also subject to ethical evaluation, the laws themselves could possibly be judged immoral and thus fail to provide a reliable guide for ethical decisions. Moreover, many of the circumstances that present ethical dilemmas are not covered by the law. For these reasons, ethics requires going beyond the view known as legalism, the idea that right and wrong are fully determined by the legal requirements that apply to a situation.

Nursing codes of ethics outline the basic moral principles that should guide the professional practice of nursing and serve to inspire moral ideals for practice. However, codes of ethics, like laws, generally offer vague statements that require interpretation in a specific case to determine what to do. According to the American Nurses Association Code of Ethics, for example, "the nurse promotes, advocates for, and strives to protect the health, safety, and rights of the patient." The dilemma that arises when these moral requirements conflict is well illustrated in the situation described in Case 1. Referring to the Code of Ethics clearly does not resolve that dilemma. Instead, a resolution calls for weighing these requirements against each other to determine what should be done.

Finally, though religions are a common source of basic ethical principles, neither ethical thinking nor ethical behavior requires a basis in a religion or in religious beliefs. What good ethical thinking does require is reflection on moral values and principles, that is, critical evaluation of the reasons that support a decision.

However, even careful ethical reasoning will not produce judgments that are beyond dispute or challenge. Some disputes can be resolved by identifying and analyzing the reasons that support different views, if individuals can agree that some reasons are more compelling. Other disagreements, though, stem from differences in values. Reasonable people may disagree about important values or the relevance of specific moral considerations and therefore arrive at different answers to ethical questions. The fact that there is no consensus concerning the answer to some ethical questions does not imply that there is no right or wrong answer but demonstrates the importance of carefully thinking through an ethical problem. Ethical decision-making should be the result of a process one is confident involves thoughtful consideration of all relevant factors and therefore produces a decision well-supported by sound reasoning.

MAKING ETHICAL DECISIONS

Good ethical decisions, like good decisions in general, result from a systematic consideration of the exact question that must be answered and the choices which could be made. Selecting a framework for thinking about the immediate problem or choosing a structure for conceptualizing the problem is an essential step in this systematic decision-making process. To illustrate the process, consider the decision to buy a house. The decision is, in practical terms, an unmanageable one if every house on the market is under consideration. In order to reach a decision, the prospective buyers will need to limit the possible options by framing the choice to incorporate the values that they decide are most important. They may frame their choice in terms of a price range and a neighborhood, or they may even limit the choices further to a particular style of house. How they frame this decision will narrow their focus to specific factors and information about a house, such as price, while other factors, such as the color of the house or the style of the kitchen, will be omitted from consideration. An important part of this whole process is deciding that all the relevant factors have been incorporated into the way the decision is framed. They can then proceed to consider the prospective purchase in terms of the framework they have chosen.

The way the decision to buy a house is framed focuses attention on specific information as most important to making that decision. Similarly, when ethical questions are confronted, how someone frames an issue determines which moral factors are considered and what information is sought about the problematic situation. Traditional moral theories can be understood as identifying different ways of framing an issue.

TRADITIONAL ETHICS

Each traditional ethical theory consists of a set of moral values and principles. These are the basis for identifying the features of a situation that are morally significant and thus provide the rationale for a decision about what is right to do. There are two commonly used approaches to ethical decision-making, one which specifies rights and a second which identifies consequences as the crucial factors to consider. Both approaches are reflected in public policy, professional decisions, and the everyday choices which individuals make.

Case 2

Oftentimes there is a conflict between family members and the patients themselves. I have a situation where the patient has a cancer diagnosis and was discharged home with home health care. Her daughter insists on making all the medical decisions for her mother and the physicians go along with this. The plan is to transfer the patient into a hospice program. But no one knows what the patient wants, because no one has asked her. **Doesn't she have a right to make these decisions herself?**

The questions raised by Case 2 can be answered by using the rights-based approach to making ethical decisions. This approach is based on the claim that specific actions are required because of the moral and legal rights of individuals. The method can be applied by asking these questions: (1) What are the moral and legal rights of each person involved? and (2) How should those rights be weighted? In cases of conflict, which rights take precedence?

Unless the patient is incompetent, or she has asked her daughter to make these decisions, the patient in this case has the fundamental right to make her own decisions about her care. This places the responsibility on others to consult her and to abide by her wishes. At the same time, the family caregivers have rights that should also be considered. For example, the patient's daughter has the right to make her own decisions about matters directly affecting her, such as whether her mother will live with her. The patient's right to decide may conflict with her daughter's rights, for example, if she were to insist on staying with her daughter against her daughter's wishes. If there is a conflict between the rights of those involved, those rights must be weighted to determine which takes precedence. From a practical perspective, negotiation and compromise will sometimes resolve a conflict between rights.

Case 3

I have a patient who is a retired nurse, a very independent woman. She is alone, with no family left at all. Though she is competent, she is not making very good choices. She doesn't have any need for skilled nursing care, but I am uncomfortable leaving her there alone. There is no food in her house, and there are hygiene issues, too, because she is not taking showers and is consequently at risk of developing skin infections. She really needs a certified nursing assistant to help with these issues, but she can't have a CNA unless there is a nurse on the case. **How can I continue to justify making these visits knowing that this patient does not have any skilled needs?**

One way to justify these visits may lie in a consideration of the consequences, which provides a second approach to ethical decision-making based on an evaluation of the costs and benefits of possible actions. The method can be applied by asking these questions: (1) What are the consequences, positive and negative, of each alternative? (2) Which consequences should be given the most weight? and (3) Which alternative offers the most benefit and the least cost overall?

All consequences, both short-term and long-term, should be considered when the results of a proposed course of action are evaluated according to this method. In Case 3, the short-term consequences of continuing to visit the patient are positive. Because the patient will have the benefit of the assistance of a certified nursing assistant, she will be safer than she would be if she were discharged from service. However, the long-term negative consequences outweigh these positive results. For example, these nursing resources could be used to address skilled nursing needs of other, sicker, patients, with greater benefit. Also, the nurse's actions, even though well-intentioned, could damage her relationship with her agency and with any other health care professionals involved in the case. Her relationship with her patient may be jeopardized, too, if the patient begins to question her trustworthiness, in light of her dishonesty on her behalf. In the final analysis, the nurse's actions cannot be justified by appealing to the results.

Case 4

My patient is an elderly man with congestive heart failure who has intractable pain. He suffers from chronic severe back pain and arthritis, and he recently broke his ankle. As a result, he is on several medications. The biggest problem is that he is on opiates, as needed, for pain control. His wife is exhausted most of the time and is having a lot of trouble coping with all of this. I think it is expecting a lot from her to have her figure out when he needs opiates. Using opiates as needed might be the ideal way to achieve pain control, but under these circumstances, I'd like to recommend that the physician reconsider this. **Should I recommend a change, even though the result would be less than what is optimum for pain management?**

Case 4 illustrates the significance of context when there are ethical issues. Traditional theories, though, maintain that general moral principles apply universally. Hence, what one person should do in a situation is the same as what any other person should do in the same circumstances. Certainly it is true that cases which are alike should be treated alike. However, neither individuals nor situations are identical. Individual people and their specific circumstances may be different in particular but ethically relevant ways. Good judgment requires knowing when such differences exist. While theories that emphasize rights and those that focus on consequences offer general guidelines, particular facts are clearly relevant. Good ethical decisions, therefore, must take into account specific features of a situation, that is, the context in which moral questions arise.

On the whole, patients have the right to the best schedule for pain medication. If the patient in this case were hospitalized, nurses would be able to administer opiates as needed to control his pain. Yet, in his particular situation, the patient must depend on his wife to decide when he needs opiates, and she is not up to the task. When these details of the patient's situation are considered, as well as rights and consequences, the nurse appears to be justified in recommending a change in medications or schedule, even though it is not the "ideal" schedule for pain control. This decision extends beyond any general principle and is tailored to the specific details of this patient in this situation.

Case 5

We had one case–a Japanese woman. She stayed in bed, drank tea, refused to eat. She stopped eating because she was very ill and did not want to be a burden to her family. She told me it was her time. **Would it be wrong for me to accept her decision to stop eating?**

The above case draws attention to the difference between the perspectives patients may have and the American cultural ideal of individualism, which depicts individuals as isolated, independent selves making decisions only for themselves. This picture does not fit the reality of the lives of most people, especially the lives of sick people in need of care. Although each patient has a distinct life history and a unique personality, together with specific desires and values that define him or her, patients are also members of families, friends, employees, and neighbors. Each person is a self involved in relationships that are valuable and that contribute substantially to who someone is as a person.

Because relationships are so important in human lives, everyday morality recognizes that people have unique obligations that single out certain people for special treatment. These obligations supersede the moral ideal to treat all people impartially. While it is important to respect all people as having equal value as human beings, it is also true that individuals have special obligations or duties to some people and not to others. Husbands and wives, for example, have specific obligations to care for each other when they are ill–obligations that they do not have to strangers. As a result, individuals' relationships, the duties that stem from their significant bonds to other people, and the consequences actions have for important relationships are crucial factors to consider when addressing ethical issues.

Accordingly, the traditional approaches to ethical decision-making must be extended to incorporate considerations about human relationships. A consequentialist approach should include the consequences for significant relationships when evaluating possible actions. This means that, in addition to appraising the costs and benefits for the individuals involved, a consequentialist approach should take into account the costs and benefits for individuals' relationships. Similarly, the rights-based approach must consider the rights deriving from relationships and the responsibilities an individual has due to important bonds to other people. Failing to recognize the significance of human relationships when framing an issue could result in overlooking what the patient would regard as decisive factors in making a choice about what to do.

In Case 5, the patient's desire to avoid burdening her family with her care is the crucial factor. Because the effects on her family are more important to her than any possible consequences for herself, this patient has decided to sacrifice her interests for the sake of what she perceives to be the interests of her family. It would be appropriate to address these matters with her, but if she is clear that she wishes to make this sacrifice, that decision should be respected.

Case 6

I did something the other day that still bothers me. One of my patients is a man with Amyotrophic Lateral Sclerosis. He asked me a question about his future with ALS just as I was ready to leave. I'm usually empathetic, but I felt I didn't have the time to deal with this then. So, I gave him a quick answer without giving him a chance to talk. I didn't live up to my own expectations and ideals. **Does that mean I am not a good nurse?**

In this case, the nurse's moral concerns revolve around basic issues about character. Having a good character involves more than just doing the right thing. It involves caring about what kind of person one is, being committed to developing the traits of a good person, and trying to do the right thing in the right way. While answering a patient's question honestly is the right thing to do, for example, the honest answer should also be delivered in a compassionate way that shows respect for a patient's concerns.

The nurse, in this instance, was not able to give as much time to addressing the patient's worries as she believes she should ideally do. Her commitment to being a good nurse is reflected in her distress about her abrupt answer. In the final analysis, nurses who strive to develop model personal characteristics in addition to the technical skills required in professional nursing, demonstrate their essential good character and exemplify the good nurse.

Some otherwise unproblematic cases may raise questions about ethical behavior that are only revealed when the situation is framed in terms of concerns about character. Thus an adequate approach to ethical decision-making must include a third way of framing the issues in addition to the rights-based approach and the consequentialist approach: What kind of person will I be if I do this? Will I be responding as a good person would respond in these circumstances?

Finally, good ethical decisions require ethical sensitivity, the capacity for recognizing ethical issues in the ordinary as well as the dramatic circumstances of human lives. Once ethical issues have been recognized, critical thinking is essential for reflecting on the way the issue is framed, assessing the possible solutions, and evaluating the reasons offered in support of each solution. Most importantly, judgment is necessary for making the decision about how to decide; in other words, choosing the best way to conceptualize a specific question about what to do, whether to assess the choices in terms of rights, consequences, or character. Judgment is also essential for deciding which factors should be given the most weight and whether an alternative solution is the best choice.

Judgment begins in the life experiences that help individuals to identify and clarify their own moral values and principles and is developed further through reflection on ethical concerns and personal values. Practice in applying ethical theory to specific cases contributes in an important way to developing judgment.

APPLYING ETHICAL THEORY: ANALYSIS OF CASE 1

Case 1 involves a patient with cancer who is dying at home. Her two sisters are staying with her to take care of her. The patient needs a colostomy but refuses to have the surgery because she doesn't think her sisters can deal with it. The issue for the nurse is whether to support the patient's decision to spare her family.

The analysis should begin with this question: Which features of this situation are ethically significant? The issues in Case 1 should be conceptualized in terms that reflect the reality that any additional burdens imposed by the patient's care will be borne by her sisters. This case does not simply involve a question of an individual's right to accept or refuse surgery; it presents the question of whether the nurse should support the patient's decision to consider only the burdens to her sisters, rather than her own health needs. To address that, the nurse could raise the question whether the patient is right in her assessment of her sisters' emotional and physical capacities. Would they really find this care too burdensome if they knew it benefits her?

The first way to frame the ethical issues in this case is to consider the moral and legal rights and responsibilities of those involved. What rights does the patient have? Does she have a right to keep information about her need for a colostomy confidential? What rights do her sisters have, if any, to information about the patient's condition? What are the nurse's responsibilities to her patient? What responsibilities does the nurse have to her patient's sisters?

Clearly, the moral and legal rights of the patient are important. Given that this patient is competent, she has the right to make the decision to accept or refuse a treatment option, based on her own ideas of what is valuable. Her sisters do not have the right to make that decision for her or to be involved in the decision-making process if she does not want their involvement.

The patient also has the right to confidentiality, which means that she can decide that health care information is to remain confidential and determine what can be shared and with whom. However, the nurse should point out the difficulty in maintaining confidentiality when her sisters are intimately involved in her care. Her sisters do have the right to any information that is necessary to providing care, but that does not include the information that the patient has refused surgery.

The nurse could explore with the patient the question of how she views her responsibilities to her sisters. Most would agree that the patient does not have the obligation to forego surgery to spare her sisters from unpleasant tasks, although she has the right to do so.

The second way to frame the issues in this case is to consider the costs and benefits. As the patient's condition worsens, the choice the patient has made to refuse the colostomy and the decision to keep this secret become increasingly problematic. These questions can be used to evaluate the consequences: What are the costs of maintaining the patient's confidentiality? Who will bear these costs? Are there significant benefits? If so, to whom? What are the consequences for the relationship between the patient and her sisters? What are the consequences for the relationship between the nurse and patient? Which consequences should be given the most weight? What is best for everyone overall?

The patient's own considerable discomfort and worsening health must be weighed against the benefits arising from respecting the patient's rights and personal values. The costs and benefits for the patient's sisters, as well as the consequences for their relationship, must also be weighed. Secrets in family relationships when patients are dying can have serious consequences, such as obstructing honest communication and interfering with emotional intimacy. The nurse should discuss these possible consequences with the patient to determine whether she remains firm in her decisions.

If the nurse decides to break confidentiality, it is likely to have substantial negative consequences for the nurse-patient relationship. Even though her intention may be to benefit the patient, violating her right to confidentiality is a serious matter.

A third way of framing the issues in Case 1 is to question what the moral ideals of nursing practice require. A final approach to this case focuses on questions about character: What do the nurse's responsibilities to her patient require? How can this nurse best meet the ideals of a good nurse? Protecting the patient's health and safety and respecting the patient's rights all satisfy the ideals of a good nurse. Since these concerns conflict in this context, this approach does not yield a final determination about what to do.

Making a decision now requires a judgment. Which moral factors are most important, rights, consequences, or character concerns? Though the consequences of both the patient's and the nurse's decisions are a matter of serious concern, the patient's right to determine what will happen to her is paramount. Individual rights may be overridden in some cases, but only when the stakes are very high, e.g., to protect people threatened by a communicable disease. In this case, the patient has the fundamental right to decide that she is willing to bear the costs to herself, for the sake of what she holds most dear, the well-being of her sisters. Therefore, the nurse should support her decision.

SUMMARY: MAKING ETHICAL DECISIONS

Context

- Which features of the particular situation are significant?

Rights

To apply the rights-based approach ask the following questions:
- What are the moral and legal rights of individuals?
- What personal relationships and responsibilities should be considered?
- If there is a conflict, which rights and responsibilities take precedence?

Consequences

To apply an approach based on consequences, ask:
- What are the costs and benefits for each person?
- What are the costs and benefits for individuals' relationships?
- Which consequences should be given the most weight?
- Which alternative is the best for everyone overall?

Character

To apply an approach focused on character, ask:
- What do moral ideals require?

Chapter 2

PATIENTS' DECISIONS, NURSES' DILEMMAS

One fundamental guiding principle in health care is that patients should make decisions for themselves. However, the decisions that patients sometimes make may seem so wrong that nurses question their role in carrying out the patient's wishes.

Case 7

One of my patients decided to live with his daughter so she could take care of him. He lets her tell him what to do. The problem is he is supposed to be on oxygen all the time, but his daughter doesn't want him on oxygen. He needs a walker; his daughter tries to get him to walk without using the walker. I talked to her until I was blue in the face. I said, "You know he needs this." She is in denial because she doesn't want her father to be sick. She told me, "He's getting better." He wants to stay with his daughter even though he seems to be risking his health. **I have to let him make these decisions for himself, don't I?**

General Issues

- **Who should make decisions for patients?**
- **What is the role of the nurse if patient safety is threatened?**
- **How should decisions be made for incompetent patients?**
- **When, if ever, may information be withheld?**

INTRODUCTION

Nurses sometimes face ethical dilemmas about the decisions of hospitalized patients, for example, when they make decisions that risk

16

their well-being. In the hospital setting, though, the decisions patients can make are usually limited to choosing to accept or reject treatments, with the result that the impact of poor judgment is generally limited to the consequences of treatment choices. Concerns about patients' decisions substantially broaden, however, when patients are cared for at home, where the range of decisions patients can make extends from treatment choices to choices about whether to live alone or with someone else, decisions about daily activities that may be consequential, and fundamental lifestyle choices. Patients may decide to live with someone who neglects them, or even someone who is frankly dangerous, or take other risks with their own health and well-being. Consequently, the dangers of the poor decisions that patients make are amplified in the home setting.

Concerns about the safety of the setting are heightened, too, when patients are cared for in their own homes, which can harbor the sort of risks that would not exist in a hospital. The physical environment may be basically unsafe, for instance, if there is substandard heating and electricity or a home lacks adequate sanitation. Patients themselves may be unable or unwilling to maintain basic standards of cleanliness. When these kinds of conditions exist, important doubts arise about whether a patient should receive nursing care at home rather than in an institution. Such concerns about patients' decisions are the source of troubling dilemmas for nurses.

WHO SHOULD MAKE DECISIONS FOR PATIENTS?

Case 8

There are elderly people who are trying so hard to stay in their own homes. I'm concerned about an elderly woman who has Parkinson's disease and osteoporosis. She ambulates by holding on to the furniture. I'm afraid she's going to get hurt. But when I said, "I hope you won't fall," she said, "I'd rather take the chance I'll break a hip. It's better than going to a nursing home." **Should I respect her decision, even though I'm not comfortable with the risks she's taking?**

For nurses, patients' decisions can create a serious conflict between the basic ethical requirements of respect for individuals' informed choices and concern for a patient's well-being when those choices demonstrate poor judgment. Respect for informed decisions is required because competent adults have the right to self-determination. This means that they have the right to make their own decisions, based on their ideas and values. This right is derived from the concept of autonomy, which means, literally, making rules for oneself. Self-determination is a fundamental right that human beings are said to have simply by virtue of being rational human beings. Respect for that right reflects the idea that human beings have dignity and intrinsic worth.

Patients thus have the right to make decisions about medical treatment, a moral right reflected in the legal requirement of informed consent. This legal requirement mandates that a patient give permission for medical treatment following disclosure of relevant information; specifically, a patient must have the capacity to make a decision, understand the information provided, and make a decision that is not coerced. When patients' decisions appear to demonstrate poor judgment, the challenge is to distinguish competent choices that satisfy the requirements for informed consent from decisions that are not informed or not voluntary, which should be questioned.

If a competent patient exercises autonomy by making a decision that is free, deliberate, and informed, that decision must be respected, unless there is a risk of harm to others. Concern for a patient's well-being alone does not justify intervention. Thus, unless there is evidence that the patient in Case 8 is incompetent, she has the right to make the choice to continue to live alone, even though she runs the risk of suffering a serious injury. In order to respect that right and at the same time promote her safety, the nurse should try to ensure that the patient understands her situation by clearly identifying the risks involved and discussing the likelihood and severity of the possible injuries risked. Finally, the nurse should review with the patient any steps she could take to make the home environment safer. For example, she could suggest contracting with an emergency response service. She should also discuss the possibility that incurring future injuries could ultimately lead to placement in a nursing home.

Nurses should document their efforts to identify risks and to communicate those risks to patients, and their attempts to assist patients in making an environment safer. Without this documentation, a nurse may be liable to disciplinary action and even legal consequences if a patient subsequently suffers harm.

WHEN A COMPETENT PATIENT'S SAFETY IS THREATENED

Case 9

I recently began caring for a seventy-five-year-old man who has just returned home from the hospital. He has serious swallowing problems, aspirates whenever he eats, and was advised that he should have a feeding tube placed. He refused, saying he is not going to give up the pleasure he gets from eating. I fully expect that one day soon I will arrive and find him dead. He is competent and well-educated about the risk he is taking. **Is there anything I should do to protect him?**

This patient may seem to need protection. From the point of view of those who put a high value on being able to extend life, he is making a very unwise decision. Health care professionals who have seen patients live a reasonably comfortable and rewarding life even with a permanent feeding tube could find it hard to understand how someone could make the choice to risk everything for the sake of being able to eat normal food. Food, however, clearly has emotional significance for many people. This patient may be unable to enjoy other pleasures, which is why he is willing to accept the risks of eating. He may also be realistic about his prospects of dying soon, even with a feeding tube, and he may have decided that he does not want to die "hooked up to machines."

The nurse's role is to initiate a dialogue with the patient to ensure that he is competent and informed about the risks he is taking. Though she may find his decision unwise, it is important to observe that individuals cannot be considered incompetent based on the fact that their choices appear unreasonable to others. The nurse can therefore counsel the patient, make recommendations about safe eating, and try to persuade him to reconsider his choices. But, because he is competent and informed, he must be allowed to live with the consequences of his own decisions.

Case 10

I have a new patient, a twenty-three-year-old war veteran who is a paraplegic. He has a very positive, almost euphoric attitude. He told me he is not going to let this condition define his life. His wife is just as positive as he is. In fact, she just accepted a promotion, which means she'll be spending more time away from home. He encouraged her to take the promotion and assured her he could take care of himself. In reality, he can't take care of himself. When I got there yesterday, I found him on the floor. He fell and couldn't get up. I think his attitude is unrealistic and dangerous. **How can I make sure that I fulfill my responsibilities to keep this patient safe?**

The patient's own optimism may constitute a danger of sorts, if he is unrealistic and does not correctly identify or appreciate the risks that are involved in trying to care for himself at home. If he has, in fact, failed to understand these risks, then his decision to remain in home health care is not an informed decision. Accordingly, the nurse's primary responsibility is to determine whether he has made an informed choice to risk his safety. She should focus renewed efforts on educating him about the risks of his situation, documenting her actions and her discussions with him. In assessing the risks and evaluating the ethical options available, the context, that is, the facts of this patient's situation, must be considered. Particular facts about the patient's home, the number of hours he is left alone, and the actions he can take if he needs assistance while his wife is out of the house, should be reviewed with the patient.

The nurse's assessment of this situation should also include another significant factor, the patient's relationship to his wife and his beliefs about his responsibility to her. His optimism may be an attempt to assure his wife that he does not need additional care and attention from her. He may be trying to protect his wife from the reality of his situation, or he may wish to ensure that she does not forfeit a career opportunity that is important to her. The risks to his own safety are perhaps far less important to him than the consequences for his relationship to his wife.

Given this, the nurse could encourage him to discuss these issues with his wife or ask his permission to talk to her about his safety. Ultimately, however, if the patient is competent and informed, he has the right to determine whether his wife is consulted about this, and he has the right to decide that he will continue to plan his life on the basis of his positive thinking, despite the possible dangers involved. Any unresolved concerns about his decisions should be reported to his physician and the agency supervisor. These actions fulfill the nurse's responsibility to act to safeguard the patient.

Case 11

I have a case where the patient is a woman with kidney disease who gets dialysis three times a week. I am seeing her for daily wound care. Her son moved in to take care of her. That's a joke. He has a long history of alcohol abuse and he is often drunk when I arrive. I think he's neglecting her, but when I tried to talk to her about it, she said he takes good care of her. **Should I do something more to protect this woman from her own son?**

Threats to a patient's safety and well-being sometimes arise from the very people who have accepted the responsibility of caring for them. Yet, an individual's right to make her own decisions includes the right to decide to live with family members or friends who act in ways that endanger her. As long as she is rational and competent, this patient can choose to have her son stay with her, even if it is not in her best interest as others would see it. Understandably, the patient may value her son's companionship above her own comfort, or she may wish to sacrifice her own well-being for the benefit of her son. That is her decision to make. The nurse could initiate conversations with the patient to explore her feelings about these matters and to assure herself that this patient is making voluntary and informed decisions. In any event, the nurse should continue to observe the situation closely and to document any instances of failure to provide adequate care. Unfortunately, she will only be able to continue to monitor the situation as long as the patient has skilled nursing needs which justify keeping her on service.

In the absence of any clear evidence of neglect or abuse by the son, the actions a nurse would be justified in taking to protect this patient are limited. If there is any sign of abuse, the nurse must make a report to the proper authorities. Failure to report elder abuse carries various penalties, dependent upon specific state statutes. In several states, the nurse would be charged with a misdemeanor and have fines imposed ranging from hundreds to thousands of dollars. In many of these states, the nurse would be subject to licensing penalties as well.

Case 12

One of my patients is on oxygen. He lives with his daughter and her boyfriend, who is a chain-smoker. The boyfriend just lost his job, so he is the primary caregiver while the daughter is at work. I tried to tell both of them that no one should be smoking near my patient because the oxygen is highly flammable.

The patient himself doesn't seem concerned and told me to quit nagging. Is there something else I should be doing to protect my patient's safety, even though he doesn't want me to do that?

Because of their expertise, nurses, physicians, and other health care professionals may believe that they are justified in restricting a patient's right to make decisions for the patient's own good. This view is called "paternalism." Paternalism would support any actions professionals take to secure a patient's safety, even when this is against the patient's own wishes. When serious safety issues arise in the home setting, paternalism may seem justified, despite the fact that it conflicts with the moral requirement to respect patient self-determination.

Paternalism is clearly justified if a patient is not competent, for incompetent patients should be protected from the consequences of their unwise decisions. Judging someone's competence, however, can be difficult. Strictly speaking, incompetence must be decided by a court, though in medical settings, informal determinations of a patient's capacity are often made by health care professionals. A legal determination of incompetence involves an assessment of orientation to time and place, ability to recognize the consequences of actions, ability to put things into logical order, and ability to make choices. If individuals are not incompetent in any of these basic ways, they are free to make decisions as unwise, risky, or idiosyncratic as they please.

Paternalism may also be justified if a person's decision is either uninformed or involuntary. For that reason, it is worth exploring why this patient continues to put himself at risk. He may not clearly understand the danger involved, or he may be reluctant to complain about the smoking. Perhaps he is afraid that his daughter will become angry or that she will evict him from her house. If that is indeed his reason for accepting the risks associated with smoking in the house, then his choice is not free and uncoerced. In the event the patient shows signs of being intimidated, the nurse should report this and thus initiate appropriate interventions.

However, if this patient is competent, and his decision is informed and voluntary, further action is not justified. He has the right to exercise autonomy and choose the circumstances in which he will live, no matter how dangerous.

Case 13

There are often safety concerns with elderly patients who live alone and refuse to be moved to a nursing facility. They may not be legally incompetent, but they're really not able to manage on their own. I have a patient with mental health problems who lives in a high-rise. He refuses to leave the apartment and refuses to go to a nursing home, despite the fact that he is not safe living alone. I'm trying to keep him safe by doing everything but moving in with him. I'm concerned that he will leave the stove on or that he will smoke and start a fire. **What am I justified in doing when a patient demonstrates such poor judgment?**

Though this patient is making poor decisions with serious consequences for his safety, he is not incompetent because he is still alert and clear about his own wishes. He may be forgetful or careless, but that in itself does not make him incompetent, nor does mental illness necessarily imply incompetence.

However, this man may pose a danger to other people who will suffer the consequences if he leaves the gas burner on and starts a fire. While his right to make decisions concerning things that affect only him must be respected in ordinary circumstances, the decisions that competent and informed individuals can make are not unlimited; when the rights and interests of others are involved, individuals' choices can be restricted on the grounds that it is required to protect others. Consequently, if there is clear evidence that he poses a danger not only to himself but also to others, then this is a situation where intervention is justified. The nurse should contact her supervisor and initiate the process.

MAKING DECISIONS FOR INCOMPETENT PATIENTS

Case 14

I have a situation with a patient who has Alzheimer's. His wife is trying to take care of him at home, but she really can't handle him. Yesterday, when I got there, he was in the tub, just sitting there. He had been in the tub for two days. He could not get out, so his wife covered him with a blanket and brought him his meals. She didn't call the rescue because she was afraid she wouldn't be able to keep him at home any more. **What should I do when the family caregiver shows poor judgment?**

When caregivers demonstrate poor judgment, nurses may doubt whether they are suited to the task of making decisions for an incompetent patient. Decisions for incompetent adults are usually made by the next of kin or a close friend on the basis of substituted judgment and authenticity. The standard of substituted judgment requires that the decision maker decide on the basis of what the patient would have wanted if competent. The patient's written statements, spoken wishes, and the values expressed to others, thus provide guidelines for surrogate decision makers. The goal is to arrive at an authentic decision, which is one that is consistent with the way the patient has lived his or her life and the values reflected by that life.

Normally, a patient's wife would have the authority to make decisions for her incompetent husband. This patient's wife presumably is doing her best to act in accordance with her husband's values and wishes by caring for him at home. However, since her limited abilities raise serious concerns about his safety and well-being, her decision to keep him home should be scrutinized.

Clearly, an important factor in such decisions is the patient's relationship to his wife, the responsibilities she believes this imposes on her, and the significance the continued relationship holds for both of them. Assuming he places great value on this relationship, the risks posed by the limitations of the patient's wife may be mitigated by the benefits of remaining at home with his wife at his side. For his wife, continuing to care for him meets the responsibilities she has to him and thus is meaningful for her. The challenge then is to find a way to support this relationship while acting to address the concerns about the patient's safety. In general, the first step is to consider ways to make it possible for him to remain safely at home as long as possible. The nurse could talk with the patient's wife to explore creative ways to deal with the difficulties of caring for him and to suggest the options available, such as a home health aide. She could help her develop a plan to deal with emergencies. She could also begin preparing his wife for the time when home health care will no longer be feasible.

Finally, the nurse must decide if this incident constitutes elder neglect. If, in fact, this is part of a larger pattern of similar incidents, it should be reported. Because the limitations of the caregiver could eventually place the patient in significant danger, this situation requires close monitoring. Currently, however, home health care agencies are not reimbursed for visits simply to monitor a situation.

Case 15

This patient is off service for a while, but then she's back again. She has coronary disease, diabetes, and peripheral vascular disease. I think she is incompetent because she is really confused. She will grimace and then, when I ask her about it, she denies she's in pain. She thinks she goes off to the office every day like she used to do, but she never leaves the house. Right now she has a black toe. She was admitted to the hospital two days ago, and the doctor wanted to amputate. But he asked her daughter, and she refused permission. Now the patient is home again and back on service. I scheduled a visit today, but her daughter met me at the door and told me, "I'll handle my mother." She wouldn't let me in. **What responsibilities do I have when the patient's daughter refuses to let me care for her mother?**

Though apparently no formal determination of incompetence has been made in this case, the patient's physician has turned to someone in the family to make decisions for the patient, as often happens. Ideally, these surrogate decisions should be made on the basis of substituted judgment. When decisions must be made for infants and others who have never been mentally competent, or in situations where there is no information about patient wishes and values, the best interest standard is used instead. This standard requires surrogates to decide based on what would be in the person's best interest.

If nurses or other professional caregivers become concerned that the next of kin is making decisions that are not based on the patient's known values and wishes, or their decisions appear to conflict with the patient's best interest, a guardian *ad litem* will be appointed by the courts as a proxy decision maker. A guardian may also be sought when there is disagreement among family members as to what the patient would have wanted to have done.

According to these standards for surrogate decision making, the patient's daughter should make decisions based on what she knows about the wishes and values her mother has, using the substituted judgment standard to determine what choices to make for her mother. It is possible, for example, that her mother would value keeping her body intact, which would justify a decision to refuse permission for an amputation. If, however, she lacks sufficient information about what her mother would have wanted in these circumstances, the daughter should make decisions based on her mother's best interest. The ethical issue arises because she has refused permission for surgery, and she has refused professional nursing care for her mother, decisions that appear to conflict with the patient's best interest.

The nurse's primary responsibility, in all professional encounters, is to act to ensure that patients receive necessary care and to advocate for patients' health and well-being. Consequently, when families interfere with care, the nurse's role is to advocate for patients' best interest. For example, she should discuss this patient's need for nursing care with her daughter, provided that the daughter will agree to speak with her. If the daughter continues to refuse her admission to the home, the nurse could attempt to reach the patient directly, perhaps with a phone call, and try to schedule another visit. Second, the nurse has the clear responsibility to report the daughter's refusal to allow her to see the patient to provide the care her physician has ordered. She should report this incident to her supervisor and the patient's physician. Finally, the daughter appears to be seriously jeopardizing her mother's well-being. This may constitute elder abuse, which must be reported to the appropriate authorities.

WITHHOLDING INFORMATION

Case 16

Doctors often leave it to the nurse to explain things to patients. Recently I started caring for a woman with three young children who has just been diagnosed with breast cancer that has metastasized to the lungs. Her physician has scheduled her for a radiation procedure with a gamma knife. I know she is not a candidate because she has multiple tumors in her lungs. I confronted her doctor: "You know she's not a candidate. Why did you schedule this?" He said, "I want to give her hope." **Should I go along with deceiving a patient in order to give her hope?**

Deceiving a patient to give her hope constitutes what is often referred to as "benevolent deception," specifically, deception which is intended to benefit the patient. This benefit is thought to justify withholding the truth. The claim of justified deception, however, conflicts with the fundamental requirement that patients be told the truth, which is essential because patients have the right of self-determination. Individuals cannot make adequate decisions for themselves if they do not have the relevant information, or if the information they have is false or biased.

The patient's right of self-determination is recognized in the legal doctrine of informed consent, which requires physicians to disclose to the patient: (1) the diagnosis; (2) the prognosis with and without the proposed treatment; and (3) the alternatives to treatment, including the risks and benefits of each alternative. There must be disclosure of any information that is *material* to a treatment decision before seeking the patient's consent.

Determining whether information is material requires analyzing two components—probability and consequences. The patient should be provided with all information that will enable her to take into account the risks of the procedure in relation to the severity of possible injury and the likelihood that the injury will occur. Everyday risks, such as the possibility of surgery-related infection, need not be disclosed.

There are two different standards that courts have used to determine a duty to disclose medical information. The first is the professional or medical community model. Under this standard of disclosure, the doctor is required to disclose only those risks that are consistent with the practice of the local community. The question is whether the physician proceeds as other competent medical professionals would in a similar situation.

The second standard is the reasonable patient standard. This standard asks what an objective, reasonable patient would consider to be relevant to the decision to consent or refuse. Doctors may not withhold information because of their own discomfort or because full disclosure might result in the patient's decision to forego treatment. Withholding the truth under such circumstances would constitute negligence, making the doctor liable for damages.

For these reasons, when a physician uses benevolent deception, the nurse's appropriate ethical response is to question the physician and express concerns about meeting the requirement for informed consent. Truly informed consent requires that patients be provided with honest alternatives, that is, options that are realistically expected to be of some benefit to the patient, which has not happened in this case. This deception compromises the possibility of informed consent and is therefore wrong.

Moreover, it is clear that nurses themselves should not deceive patients, even in order to give them hope, and, if asked direct questions, nurses should not lie to patients. Volunteering information, however, could create a conflict with the physician. The nurse could instead suggest that the patient ask the doctor for more exact information about her condition and prognosis.

This case demonstrates the integral, though sometimes unacknowledged, role nurses often play in informed consent. Patients expect them to explain what physicians have left unexplained, to clarify and interpret what they have been told, and to answer the questions they may hesitate to ask their physicians. This role is enhanced in home health care because patients see doctors less frequently than when they are hospitalized.

Case 17

One of my patients is an elderly woman who broke her collar bone. Her daughter told me that the doctor said her mother also had an aneurysm and won't live long. The mother is very nervous and easily upset, so her doctor has decided to tell her nothing about this. Her daughter agrees and insists that I promise I won't say anything to the patient or to the other nurses. She's afraid her mother will find out. **When is it permissible to withhold information from a competent patient? Is it ever permissible to withhold information from other health care professionals?**

There are three exceptions to legal rules regarding informed consent and disclosure of information to patients. The first is in an emergency situation when the patient is unconscious or otherwise incompetent to make a decision and immediate treatment is required. That is, the harm from failure to treat is imminent and outweighs the harm likely to be brought about by the treatment itself. In these situations, courts have agreed that physicians can act without informed consent as long as treatment is in accordance with standard emergency practice. Going further, some courts have held that informed consent is implied in all emergency situations.

The second exception to the doctrine of informed consent occurs when a competent patient waives the right to receive medical information. A waiver is the voluntary and intentional relinquishment of a known right. A competent patient, for example, could decide she does not want to be informed of the details of a medical condition and direct that medical information be disclosed instead to a family member, thereby waiving her right to full disclosure.

The third exception, relevant in this case, involves the notion of therapeutic privilege. This concept acknowledges that, at times, disclosure of medical information renders patients incapable of rational decision-making, complicates or hinders treatment, or perhaps even poses the risk of psychological damage to the patient. Therapeutic privilege is a controversial exception to the requirement to disclose information, however, and the law is unclear as to its scope. As such, this "privilege" must be carefully circumscribed. Nurses should therefore scrutinize any claims of therapeutic privilege and clarify with physicians the basis for considering information harmful if therapeutic privilege is claimed. The exception is justified only if there are compelling reasons for believing disclosure will harm the patient. Otherwise, nurses should advocate for truthful disclosure.

Nonetheless, the exception of therapeutic privilege appears to justify withholding the diagnosis from this patient, based on the daughter's assessment of the emotional and psychological state of her mother. This will mean, however, that the patient will be denied the opportunity to address any "unfinished business" before she dies, which presumably would be important to her. The significance of this should be discussed with her daughter to help her evaluate her decisions concerning her mother.

Should a nurse withhold this information from other nurses? The answer is an unequivocal "no." A nurse would be guilty of unprofessional conduct if she filed a false report or record, or if she failed to furnish appropriate details about a patient's nursing needs to other nurses involved in providing continuing nursing services.

ANALYSIS OF CASE 7

Case 7 describes the situation of a patient who wants to live with his daughter despite the fact that her actions appear to be risking his health. The question is whether patients should be allowed to make their own decisions when their safety is significantly threatened as a result.

Generally, a competent individual's rights are the prevailing considerations in such a situation. Competent adults have the right to self-determination, which includes the right to make decisions about medical treatment. Even life-saving treatment can be rejected by a competent adult who has made a voluntary, informed decision. This patient therefore has the right to make his own choices, including the decision to live with his daughter and accept her judgments about his care.

The nurse's moral dilemma in Case #7 arises from conflicting oblig-ations. She has a commitment to protect patients' moral and legal rights, but she also has an ethical and professional responsibility to promote a patient's health. When patients exercise poor judgment, refuse necessary treatments, or in other ways accept risks to their health and well-being, the expected results of their unwise decisions seem to require action to protect them, but that would violate respect for their right to make their own decisions.

The traditional approaches to ethical decision-making appear to force a choice between respect for rights and consideration of conse-quences. But, as this kind of case illustrates, focusing exclusively on either rights or consequences is an inadequate method for resolving these issues. Attending only to the patient's right to decide whatever he chooses appears to mean that others have to stand by while he makes decisions that will result in serious harm to himself. On the other hand, focusing exclusively on the consequences of his decision may lead to an illegitimate form of paternalism. Paternalistic interfer-ence with a competent patient's right to decide, on the grounds that it is for his own good, cannot be justified.

The key to resolving the nurse's moral conflict, the question of how to advocate for the patient's rights and, at the same time, fulfill the commitment to the patient's health and safety, lies in extending the analysis of the particular situation to include considerations of signifi-cant ethical factors in addition to rights and consequences. In Case 7, that means that the nurse must include consideration of the patient's relationship with his daughter. He has chosen to live with his daughter and she in turn has accepted the responsibility for his care. Clearly, this relationship is very important to the patient, both emotionally and physically. The nurse should thus take into consideration the conse-quences for that relationship as she tries to determine what to do. Supporting the patient's decision to continue living with his daughter will presumably enhance their relationship. If the nurse continues to address the daughter's denial, and tries to minimize the negative con-sequences by suggesting additional safety measures, the patient's rela-tionship to his daughter will benefit, and the risks to his safety will diminish. On the other hand, if she attempts to interfere with the patient's decision out of concern for his health and safety, she will be forced to argue that the daughter's care harms her father. The possibly destructive consequences for the family relationship do not justify this response in this circumstance. Considering the effects on the patient's relationships clarifies the decision: the nurse should support the patient's decision to live with his daughter, despite the risks.

The nurse should also support the patient's right to give informed consent for any medical treatments. Her continuing efforts to provide information and explain the risk of neglecting treatment are a way to ensure that the father's decisions are informed. In this way she acknowledges the patient's decision to accept risks, while at the same time she is doing all she can to protect his safety and reduce the dangers.

ETHICAL CRITERIA

- The competent patient has a right to exercise autonomy, that is, make free, deliberate, and informed decisions.
- The patient has a right to truthful information.

PRACTICAL STRATEGIES

When the patient lives alone:

- Educate the patient about any risks involved.
- Determine alternatives to risky situations.
- Act to make the environment safer.

When patients live dangerously:

- Ensure that the patient is competent and that decisions are fully informed.
- Explain risks and alternatives.
- Act to diminish the risks.
- Attempt to persuade the patient to avoid risks.
- Intervene when the risks involve others.

When patients are unrealistic:

- Educate patients about the nature and risks of their situation.
- Ask permission to raise the issue with the family caregiver.

When patients' families create risks:

- Educate patients and family members about the risks.
- Ask the patient's permission to raise the issue with others.
- Suggest actions to diminish the risks.
- Report to the supervisor when the risk seems unacceptable.

When patients are incompetent:

- Assure that there is a competent caregiver.
- Advocate for decisions that agree with the patient's known wishes and values.
- Contact supervisors and outside agencies when caregivers abuse or neglect the patient.

When physicians use benevolent deception:

- Discuss the reasons for withholding information with the physician.
- Advocate for truthful disclosure.
- Encourage the patient to ask questions.

When families withhold information:

- Explore what the patient wants to know through questioning.
- Answer the patient's questions honestly.
- Educate the family about the patient's right to truthful information.

When therapeutic privilege is cited as a reason for withholding information:

- Discuss with the physician the reasons the information is considered harmful.
- Advocate for disclosure of as much truthful information as possible.
- Communicate truthfully with all members of the health care team.

Chapter 3

THE ROLE OF THE FAMILY

Nurses caring for patients at home face ethical questions about the role family caregivers should have when decisions are made, particularly when family decisions appear to jeopardize a patient's health or safety.

Case 18

Families have to be involved in home health care, but it doesn't always work out well. I am caring for a man who had a devastating stroke. His son moved him into his house to care for him. My patient complained to me that his son is not bathing him often enough or feeding him regularly. Then he started to cry and said he didn't want to do anything to upset his son. Even though he clearly needs nursing care, I just learned that his son wants to stop the home health care visits. **Should his son be the one to make these decisions?**

General Issues

- **What is the role of the family in decision making?**
- **What is the nurse's responsibility when families jeopardize the patient's well-being?**
- **What should nurses do when family disagreements affect the patient's care?**
- **What are the limits of obligations to caregivers?**

INTRODUCTION

The decisions patients make and the care they receive may be profoundly influenced by their families, but this influence is limited in some ways if patients are hospitalized. Though issues about families and their proper role in decisions can arise in that setting, families cannot ordinarily deny the hospitalized patient's ethical and legal right to make decisions nor interfere directly with the professional care the patient receives. However, patients are not as insulated from their families' influence in the home setting where families usually have a substantial role in providing care.

Family caregivers who are devoted, competent, and responsible constitute the ideal for home health care. Nevertheless, a family's response to sickness and the responsibilities of caring for someone who is ill or dying can vary greatly. In truth, some family caregivers may actually be psychologically and emotionally incapable of providing the intimate, personal care required. At times families are also intolerant of the changes that poor health can cause in a loved one. Moreover, all the unresolved conflicts inherent in family relationships can be exacerbated by the stress of illness. Adult children, for example, may harbor resentments that complicate their involvement in caring for their parents. Patients, too, respond in different ways to their illnesses. Some find it particularly difficult to accept help from their families, while others demand their unstinting attention and care, placing an unreasonable burden on their caregivers. As a result, this is a setting where nurses often struggle with ethical concerns about the role of the family and their professional and moral responsibilities to family caregivers.

THE FAMILY'S ROLE IN DECISION MAKING

Case 19

One of my patients is a woman who has no mobility from the waist down. She can't get out of bed to her wheelchair without assistance. Three weeks ago she was diagnosed with a very serious decubitus. I see her five days a week for the dressing changes she needs for the bed sores. Her husband washes her and changes the dressing in the morning before he goes to work and again when he gets home. He doesn't get her out of bed, though. She's in bed all day when what she needs is to be up for an hour, back in bed an hour, then up again. There are three adult children living nearby, but they have not helped at all. Her husband is burning out. He can't keep her at home like she wants and continue to work full time at the job he has. **What role should I encourage a family to take when decisions like this have to be made?**

Because family caregivers often have a critical role in home health care, patients' decisions, such as the decision this woman has made to remain at home, will have a definite impact on them. The integral role of the family thus raises important issues about how these decisions should be made and whether families should be involved. Even for competent patients who are capable of making decisions, there are different ways in which decision making can be conceptualized.

The most commonly accepted model today is shared decision making. Though it usually refers to the doctor-patient relationship, it can be extended in the home health care setting to family-patient relationships. Shared decision making may be contrasted to individualistic decision-making, where patients are left on their own to decide for themselves, considering only their own interests. Clearly, the moral and legal requirements for informed consent appear to assume that patients' decisions are purely unilateral and individual. The assumption is that, when a decision is necessary, patients think through the issues independently and reach a decision. Patients are thus free to choose among different treatments, or to refuse any and all treatment, informed by medical information and reaching conclusions based solely on their own set of values.

There is a problem with this model. Though some decisions do seem to have implications only for an individual patient, most decisions will have an impact on other people, especially in the home health care setting. For example, if a patient decides to reject transfer to a rehabilitation center or nursing home, this means, in effect, that someone must be willing and able to continue to care for the patient at home. This kind of decision could force a family member who is already overwhelmed by other responsibilities, or perhaps in poor health, to accept this obligation. That imposes an unfair burden on the family member. Obviously, an individual's right to choose cannot include the right to make such impossible demands on others. Further, given that all individuals are involved in relationships with several other people, a totally individualistic model of decision-making does not reflect the reality of people's lives.

The model of shared decision making, on the other hand, does reflect the reality of individuals' involvement in relationships and provides a way to make decisions that takes into account the interests and rights of others, as well as recognizing the patient's ethical and legal right to make medical choices. Shared decision making involves both collaboration and compromise. In collaborative decision-making, patients retain their central role in making final decisions for themselves but reach their conclusions after consultation with their families. This process is particularly useful when patients are unsure about their own wishes. Family members participate by sharing their own views about what it would be best for the patient to do and contribute ideas that could aid the patient in reaching a decision. At the end of the process, the patient makes a decision based on the discussion.

Consider, for example, an elderly patient who must decide whether to continue to live with a relative, as his family wants him to do, or agree to be placed in a nursing home. He knows his family will not be able to provide the same level of care that he would receive in an institution where professional staff is present. He is aware, consequently, that he is risking his health to some extent if he remains at home. If he is not sure what to do, he could consult with his family and they could discuss the possibilities together. Gradually, through sharing their ideas, they should be able to clarify his options and his wishes. They may establish that he really wants to stay at home, despite the limitations that involves, and they could then conclude that it is a reasonable choice for him. Although it remains his decision, they have come to the decision together.

On this model, patients see themselves not as isolated individuals, but as members of a family that operates as a community. They recognize family relationships as important to their thinking. The limitation of this model is that it works only when there are good relationships among those involved.

Compromise decision making is a process in which competent patients who have clear ideas about what they want are willing to shape their decisions in response to the wishes of others. Individuals and family members begin this process by sharing their ideas of what they each want to happen. Through negotiation and compromise, each is persuaded to yield in some way. The patient is able to make a decision that is as close to his or her original wish as is practically feasible, but that still responds to the concerns of others.

Compromise decision making could be utilized in Case 19. Though the patient wants to remain at home, her husband is not able to provide care during the day unless he takes time off from work. In addition, he has been attempting to care for her without any help from their adult children. To address the problems this has created, the patient, her husband and children might compromise in the following way. The husband and children could agree to share the daily task of caring for the patient, each providing a few hours of care one or two days a week, with a promise to rethink this if the arrangement imposes too great a burden on any of them. The patient's children thus accept some responsibility for their mother's care and her husband agrees to take more time off from work than he would like. The advantage of this kind of decision making is that it recognizes the patient as the final decision maker but allows for input from others and seeks a solution that works for everyone. The disadvantage is that in some cases, the individuals may be so far apart or so adamant in their original positions that compromise is impossible.

Though decision making for home health care patients ideally utilizes shared decision making, nurses should help families understand that, from both a moral and legal perspective, the patient is the final decision maker. Nevertheless, patients should be encouraged to weigh the impact their individual decisions will have on others.

Case 20

I have a really difficult case right now, a young woman who is dying from colon cancer. Her husband hardly leaves her side. He complains she's sleeping all the time, and he wants to spend time with her. He doesn't want us increasing her morphine even though she's in pain. **Should he have the right to decide what medications she receives?**

Though this patient is not now competent to decide for herself whether she receives increased pain medication, any decisions that are made on her behalf should respect her prior expressions of wishes concerning treatment. If, in past conversations or past experiences with illness, she expressed her feelings about receiving large amounts of pain medication even if it would sedate her to the point of unconsciousness, then it is possible to use the standard of substituted judgment to make the decision she would make if she could. This is a standard that is recognized by the courts in cases where there is disagreement among family members about treatment for a patient who has become incompetent.

Without any information concerning her wishes, treatment decisions should be made on the basis of the best interest standard. Unfortunately, there can be disagreement about what is in someone's best interest. Some individuals argue that the quality of life is most important, whereas others believe the opposite, that extending the length of life is always in an individual's best interest.

An alternative standard that is sometimes invoked is the reasonable person standard. What would a reasonable person in these circumstances choose for herself? This may also be subject to disagreement, for what seems reasonable to some may not seem reasonable to others. Further, there may be cultural differences that determine what individuals believe to be reasonable. These standards, therefore, must be used with careful attention to the details of a case. Calculating this patient's best interest, or what is reasonable, requires attention to the costs and benefits associated with end of life care, and her need for relief from pain, as well as addressing her particular situation and the effect of any decisions on her family relationships.

Under the best of circumstances, the patient and her husband would have discussed the choices that need to be made for her and could have used shared decision making to reach mutually agreeable conclusions about her care at the end of life. If that process had resulted in her decision to stay conscious for as long as possible, her husband's actions would be reasonable. Otherwise, the husband's insistence that his wife be conscious violates her presumed best interest and should be resisted.

It is possible that he does not realize how close she is to death and how much pain she is experiencing. Given this possibility, the nurse should focus on educating the patient's husband about the reality of the situation and attempt to motivate decisions based on compassion for the patient. This might lead to a satisfactory resolution. If necessary, the nurse could contact her supervisor at the agency with any concerns she has about this family member's decisions concerning medications. Discussions with the agency's ethics committee, if it has one, would also be helpful.

Recent studies show that many patients at the end of life do not receive sufficient pain medication and spend their last days experiencing significant pain. There is consensus that, unless a patient, when competent, chose to refuse or minimize pain relief, sufficient medication should be administered.

WHEN FAMILIES JEOPARDIZE THE PATIENT'S WELL-BEING

Case 21

I have a patient whose wife second guesses the doctors. She tries to control everything that happens. I found out she had doubled up on the Lasix, which affects his potassium levels. She said, "Don't worry, I have potassium pills I'm giving him, too." I have tried to explain that her interference with his medications may be harmful, but she says she knows him better than we do. I know she is doing what she thinks is best for him, still it's dangerous for her to make these changes. **How can I guarantee that the patient gets the care he needs?**

Even families that are well meaning sometimes make questionable decisions or interfere with a patient's care, based on their assumption that they know the patient better than the doctors do. Because families presumably have reasons for making their own changes in a plan of care, nurses should initiate a discussion of these decisions with caregivers to determine what led to the changes. When a family caregiver adjusts or omits a medication, for example, it is likely that he or she has noticed some difference or side effect that led to this decision. Caregivers should be encouraged to bring those changes to the attention of the nurse so that the nurse can assess the need for a change in medication or dosage and contact the physician if necessary.

This patient's wife appears to be sincerely concerned about his well-being. Thus, effective teaching about the dangers of adjusting his medications should help to resolve the problem in this case. The patient should also be fully informed of the medications and dosages that his physician has prescribed and encouraged to contact the nurse if he has some questions about the medicine he is taking. Any concerns about the patient's safety must of course be reported to the agency supervisor and the patient's physician.

Case 22

I can't believe what some families do. One of my patients is a very wealthy elderly man. He came on the service for wound care. Medicare pays for that. He also has round-the-clock nursing care he's paying for himself. His nephew, however, has power of attorney over his financial affairs. After the first bill arrived and he saw how much it cost, his nephew decided his uncle just needs the daytime nurse covered by Medicare. Now he has his friends coming in to care for his uncle. He said he's afraid his uncle will run out of money. That will never happen! I know the uncle won't say anything. **Is this any of my business? Should I keep my concerns to myself?**

Home health care nurses have the professional responsibility to determine when the behavior of families justifies intervening on behalf of patients, which implies that family decisions limiting nursing care are a legitimate concern. This patient, of course, has the right to decide to reduce or eliminate nursing services himself, as long as he is competent and fully aware of his medical condition.

Here, however, it is not clear that the patient has freely agreed to be cared for by his nephew's friends instead of professional caregivers. It is evident that he is dependent on his nephew, who has the power of attorney and is in a position to make the decisions that allow this elderly man to remain in his own home. This raises the possibility that the uncle's tacit acceptance of this change is not fully voluntary. Given this possibility, the nurse should advise the nephew that the patient has the right to make these decisions. She should also talk to the patient about his wishes. He may be willing to accept less nursing care and comfort in exchange for being able to remain in his own home. As long as he has freely chosen to accept his nephew's decision, the patient's right to self-determination has not been violated. The nurse should ensure that he understands the consequences of that decision.

The possibility of elder abuse and neglect must also be considered in such cases. Elder abuse and neglect includes both physical and emotional harm, comprised of physical assault, verbal and sexual abuse, isolation, confinement, and financial exploitation. Such crimes against elders, like crimes against children, are deemed worthy of special consideration because the victims are considered more vulnerable and have a greater degree of dependence. Therefore, they warrant additional protection through the coercive power of the law. The problem is that after the nurses have been discharged, there may be no one in a position to monitor the patient's condition.

WHEN FAMILY DISAGREEMENTS AFFECT
THE PATIENT'S CARE

Case 23

Families can sometimes sabotage the plan of care we have. One of my patients is a widower who has lived alone for years. His daughter lived out of state, but she moved back home when he got sick. He had already decided that he didn't want any further treatment. His daughter refuses to accept that. She calls him a "coward" and a "quitter" for not fighting. He told me not to do anything about this, just to "let his daughter be." **Should I try to get her to accept her father's decision or let them work it out?**

As an advocate for the patient's right to self-determination, nurses should promote the family's acceptance of a patient's decisions, including the decision to forego further treatment at the end of life. Family conflicts about patient decisions could be addressed by explaining the patient's ethical and legal right to choose and offering to facilitate a family meeting to discuss disagreements, if the patient consents. When family disagreements are significant, the nurse should encourage shared decision making as a process that would respect the patient's right to make medical choices but also attempt to accommodate the family's feelings about the patient's illness and their concerns as family caregivers.

Shared decision making, however, will not be successful when family disagreements about end-of-life treatment appear to be intractable. The nurse's concern then is protecting the patient's mental and physical well-being, for such family conflicts will most likely increase the level of tension and stress when patients are dying at home. Most importantly, significant disagreements can damage family relationships at a time when they are most valuable for patients and families. Rejecting a patient's difficult choices and calling a dying patient a "quitter" because he has decided to forego additional treatment could have a devastating effect on the patient and result in emotional isolation and mistrust. The nurse should attempt to protect the patient from this mistreatment and encourage a more nurturing relationship between father and daughter, for the patient's sake. With the patient's permission, the nurse should discuss with the daughter the reality of the situation and attempt to lead her to an acceptance that will support her father's decision. She should also identify the harm the daughter is doing with her rejection of his decisions. However, if the patient does not agree to allow this discussion, the nurse should leave it to them to work out on their own. It is important to note that nurses cannot discuss the patient's health without permission, even with family members, because of a patient's right to confidentiality.

Case 24

One of my patients wants so much to please her family, she does not communicate honestly when they are there. She's declining, but the family is in denial. They are very protective. They hover around her and prevent her from talking privately to me. When we have had time alone, she has been reviewing her life. I don't think the family wants to let her do that. **How can I help the patient face dying when her family won't allow it?**

The conflict between this patient and her family is silent and unacknowledged, but it is the source of real quandaries for nurses who are prevented from acting in the patient's best interest. Resolving such quandaries requires attention to the patient's wishes and the value the patient places on family relationships.

Patients sometimes make decisions that benefit their families, yet at the same time harm their own interests. Some patients, for instance, want their families to be able to deny what is happening when they are seriously ill, because they think this makes it easier for the family. As a consequence, unfortunately, they relinquish any opportunity to discuss with their families matters that are important to them when they are dying.

Though this patient could probably benefit if the family were not in denial about the reality of her situation, she should be the one to determine whether the nurse discusses this matter with anyone in the family. The nurse could offer to talk with the family for her, with her permission, or offer to be present to help her broach the subject with them herself. This would free them to talk to each other about any important issues, if they wish to do so.

If the patient still wishes to allow the family to deny how sick she is, then the nurse should respect that wish. Her only option, then, is to attempt to arrange sufficient private time for the patient to have the opportunity to ask her questions about dying and express her feelings. This must be done in a way that does not upset the patient's family or interfere with the patient's relationship with her family.

Case 25

I am caring for a woman who is seriously ill with ovarian cancer. Her physicians have just begun very aggressive chemotherapy treatment that has a small chance of success. When I am there, she confides that she really just wants to stop. She understands what will happen, but she is so weak and tired, she just wants it to be over. Her daughter visits every week and urges her mother to keep going, so she does. **How do I know what to do when a patient is ambivalent?**

It is understandable that patients who face difficult decisions about cancer treatment may have a change of heart about what they want to do. They may say one thing one day but change their mind the next day, or say different things to different people. Some patients are so eager to please their families that it is difficult to know if they are making authentic decisions, that is, decisions that reflect their own wishes and values.

When patients frequently change their minds, it is tempting to interpret this as a reason to suspect diminished competence. However, there is another way to interpret indecision or conflicting statements from patients. The woman in this case has true ambivalence about continuing chemotherapy, an ambivalence that is the result of being caught between two deeply-held values. She wants to end what has come to feel like a life with more pain and suffering than positive moments, but she also wants to show her love for her daughter, which explains why she continues to accept the treatment. For a woman who has been socialized to sacrifice herself for the sake of others, a decision based simply on her own interests may seem to her selfish and unacceptable.

From a moral perspective, it is important to observe that helping patients preserve significant relationships is an ethical consideration on a par with acknowledging the right to self-determination and weighing the consequences of decisions to determine what is right to do. The nurse can support this mother in her dedication to her daughter, while acknowledging the conflict she feels. The mother may benefit from referral to a professional counselor who will help her understand the dynamics of the mother-daughter relationship and clarify her feelings and values. This will help her to recognize which decision she truly wants to make. If anyone questions the patient's competency due to her vacillations about treatment, the nurse could suggest this analysis of the situation, as one in which the mother is ambivalent because she has sincerely-held but conflicting values.

Case 26

> Some families really get in the way. I have a patient with esophageal cancer. She says the care that she is getting is fine, but her daughter hates us. The sicker her mother gets, the harder it is to deal with her daughter. None of the nurses want to go there. When I got there yesterday, she met me at the door and shouted, "She's dying. What the hell are you going to do about it?" I want out, but I think the agency will drop her if one more nurse quits this case. **What should I do?**

Despite the best efforts of nurses, conflicts may arise between nurses and families that make it difficult to maintain the appropriate professional relationships that are essential as a basis for providing nursing care. Moreover, the subsequent tension will add to the stress of serious illness and adversely affect the patient. In the event that conflicts with the family affect a patient's health, a nurse's primary obligation is to act as an advocate for the patient. She should attempt to discuss the situation with this patient's daughter and to explain the harm her behavior causes her mother. However, the nurse's own ability to help is limited, given the daughter's hostility to her. One course of action would be to recommend counseling to help the daughter control her feelings of hostility, since her expressions of anger are a recognized stage of the grieving process. A social worker could help her understand the impact on her mother and help her develop appropriate coping skills.

Finally, no one is expected to work under abusive conditions. Nurses can justifiably withdraw from a case when conflicts with the family jeopardize their ability to provide nursing care, assuming that they follow the appropriate steps in accordance with agency policy and state law. Because several nurses have already quit the case, the agency is unlikely to want to continue to keep this patient on service. Nonetheless, this nurse does not have a special obligation to tolerate hostility and to continue caring for the patient. If she decides to continue on this case, her actions are supererogatory, that is, above and beyond what is morally required.

Case 27

I don't understand families who can't put aside their differences when someone is sick. It is really tough when they don't get along. I have a Lupus patient who wants to see her mother, but her husband refuses to allow it. He's never forgiven her mother for something that happened years ago. I want to help her, but I don't want to get in the middle of a family feud. **How far does my responsibility to my patient extend?**

A nurse could justifiably consider this concern to lie outside her professional duty to provide skilled nursing care. As an advocate for her patient, nonetheless, she may believe she has a moral responsibility to address a situation that is causing considerable distress for her patient.

One way to approach the question about her responsibilities would be to reflect on the behavior that would best fulfill her professional ideals. An important objective for nurses is to ease the suffering of patients. She may be able to realize the ideal of a caring nurse by responding to the patient's emotional suffering, but she should obviously only take action with the patient's permission. First, she could talk with the patient's husband to impress on him the significance of the situation and how important it is for the patient to see her mother. Second, if the patient requests it, she could consider contacting the patient's mother herself. Whatever action she does take, she must weigh carefully the possible consequences for the patient's relationship to her husband.

THE LIMITS OF OBLIGATIONS TO CAREGIVERS

Case 28

Sometimes we get assigned to cases and it turns out that the caregiver needs more help than the patient. I have an Alzheimer's patient who becomes difficult whenever his wife is in the same room. She is in her eighties, but when he starts acting up, she needs to leave the house. She'll drive around for hours at a time. Her children want to put him in a nursing home. She told me she can't do that because "I took a vow." She can't cope, though she refuses to admit it. **How do I balance my responsibilities to the caregiver and to the patient?**

While nurses are, first and foremost, patient advocates, home health care nurses do have an obligation to act on behalf of caregivers if their health or safety is endangered. Generally, every person has a moral obligation to prevent harm to others when it is possible to do so without substantial sacrifice or great difficulty. Accordingly, the nurse should discuss frankly with the patient's wife the risk to her own health and well-being if the patient remains at home. Nevertheless, she may prefer to take that risk rather than place her husband in a nursing home. If that is the case, the nurse could seek additional services, such as respite care, to help her cope with the burden of caring for her husband.

This responsibility to respond to concerns about a caregiver must be weighed against the nurse's duty to advocate for patient safety and well-being. If the limitations of the caregiver pose a risk of harm to the patient, then the nurse has a clear obligation to take the appropriate action to protect him. She should explain the hazards and urge his wife to rethink the decision to care for him at home. She should also contact his physician to evaluate the need for placement in a nursing facility, even if his wife objects. Though concerns about family caregivers are important, nurses' responsibilities to them are limited by their primary responsibility, the obligation to act as an advocate for the patient.

Families are often supportive allies for health care professionals, yet they can sometimes present obstacles to good nursing care. Nurses must achieve a delicate balance between respecting caregivers for the important role they play and advocating for patients who are very dependent on the ability and goodwill of others.

ANALYSIS OF CASE 18

Case 18 involves an elderly patient whose son is his caregiver. While the care his son is providing is sometimes inadequate, the patient does not want to upset his son by questioning his actions. However, when his son appears ready to discharge the home health care nurses, the nurse faces the issue of the role the son should play in these decisions for his father.

Certainly the patient's son should not usurp his father's right to make decisions about care, based on his right of self-determination.

This patient ultimately has the right to make the decision to live with his son, despite the substandard care he provides, or, instead, to move out of his son's home, perhaps to a nursing home. The nurse can help the patient think through what is right for him by spelling out the consequences, that is, the costs and benefits of these two choices. She can help him to think about what will happen to him if he agrees to stop the nursing visits. She can also guide him through a consideration of the consequences of a break with his son and the adjustment to life in a nursing home. In the end, he may decide that his family relationship is most important and that he will accept his son's decisions, which is his right. That is, he can relinquish the right to make his own medical decisions.

Ideally, father and son would have utilized a shared decision-making process to reach a decision that addresses the concerns of both of them. Though a nurse should advance a patient's right to decide, in this particular context, it is essential that she is also sensitive to the patient's concern about his relationship with his son. The nurse can respond to her concern about the son's neglect by attempting to re-educate him about his father's health care needs and the possible dangers of his own inattention to his father. At the same time, she must be careful to protect the father's confidences and avoid antagonizing the son, because of the effect that could have on the family relationship.

Finally, if she believes the patient's health and safety are endangered, she must report this situation to her supervisor and the appropriate agencies. Nevertheless, she should not pursue this matter with outside authorities unless there is some evidence of serious neglect or abuse.

ETHICAL CRITERIA

- Competent patients have the right to make their own decisions.
- Competent patients may voluntarily relinquish that right to someone else.

PRACTICAL STRATEGIES

When the patient's decisions significantly affect the family:

- Encourage the patient to recognize how decisions affect the family.
- Promote shared decision making.

When the family interferes with the plan of care:

- Educate the family about the reasons for the prescribed plan of care.
- Acknowledge and support the family's efforts to care for the patient.
- Advocate for the patient's best interest by contacting the supervisor and the ethics committee if necessary.

When the family's motives and decisions raise concerns:

- Ask a competent patient's permission before raising these issues with the family.
- Encourage the family to respect a competent patient's wishes.
- Ensure the patient's safety needs and best interest are served.
- Provide information on resources and support services for families.
- Contact the appropriate authorities when abuse and neglect are suspected.

When disagreements affect patient care:

- Advocate for patient rights.
- Recommend shared decision making.
- Engage in conflict resolution with the family.
- Encourage family counseling.

When the family caregiver cannot cope:

- Inform the caregiver about alternatives and support services.
- Take appropriate action if the caregiver's limitations pose a risk of harm to the patient or caregiver.

Chapter 4

SAFEGUARDING SECRETS, PROTECTING PRIVACY

Home health care patients sometimes keep important information about their health secret from their families, even though revealing that information may be to their benefit. Nurses then confront an ethical conflict between acting to promote the patient's health and recognizing patient rights to confidentiality.

CASE 29

One of my HIV patients is a forty-two-year-old male. He is so dysfunctional that he is not able to work. Even though his HIV medications are paid for by a state-subsidized AIDS program, the program doesn't cover the antidepressants or the pain medications he needs. He refuses to let me contact his parents for help because they don't know he is HIV-positive. **Should I talk to them anyway so he gets his medications?**

General Issues

- **Who should have access to information about patients?**
- **When is a nurse justified in breaching confidentiality?**
- **How far should nurses go to protect their patients' privacy?**
- **What responsibilities does a nurse have to protect family privacy?**

INTRODUCTION

Hospitalized patients can assert control over personal medical information and thus maintain secrecy about their health if they wish to do so. They can expect that families and others will not have access to their hospital records and that health care professionals will not share medical information unless it is medically necessary or patients explicitly give permission. This is in sharp contrast to the situation in home health care where there are not many secrets about patients' health. Families have an opportunity to gain access to confidential medical information from any medical record or travel chart that is kept in the home. This is a special concern when sensitive personal matters are documented. Further, families often fail to understand the ethical requirement to respect patient confidentiality and presume that nurses should disclose to them whatever medical information they seek about a patient.

When they care for patients in their own homes, nurses inadvertently learn personal, nonmedical information about patients and their families. They observe their patients' lifestyles and personal habits, their financial circumstances, family relationships, and family "secrets." The ethical question is the extent to which private, nonmedical information should be protected and when, if ever, otherwise confidential information should be disclosed to others.

ACCESS TO INFORMATION ABOUT PATIENTS

Case 30

I'm caring for a patient who has been a very popular member of the staff at the agency. She is currently out on a medical leave. Everyone knows I'm her nurse. When I get back to the office from my home visit, everyone asks: "Oh, you saw Joanne today. How's she doing?" **Can I tell them anything?**

Though it may seem harmless to answer that question about how a patient is doing, it would normally be a violation of confidentiality. From a legal point of view, confidentiality is protected by privileged communication statutes. The nurse-patient relationship, like the physician-patient relationship, is a confidential one. This means that nurses must refrain from discussing patients with third parties, regardless of their benign intentions. A nurse who breaches confidentiality commits a tort, which is a violation of an individual's legal rights. Depending on the jurisdiction in which the complaint is filed and the circumstances involved, a nurse could be charged with breach of confidence, breach of contract, or invasion of privacy for revealing confidential medical information, including the very fact that an individual is her patient.

Staff members, friends, and neighbors who are familiar with an individual's medical situation may expect a nurse to answer questions about a patient, assuming that their established relationship and benevolent interest justify responding to their request for information. A close relationship to a patient, however, does not provide a sufficient rationale for disclosing personal medical information. Similarly, unless a health care professional is directly involved in caring for a patient, which justifies sharing information relevant to the patient's treatment and well-being, health care professionals have no claim to further information than what they may inadvertently glean from working in the health care facility or agency that is caring for the patient. The American Nurses Association Code of Ethics identifies the nurse's duty to maintain the confidentiality of all information received from or about the patient, whether the communication is oral, written, or electronic, and to share relevant data only with those health care professionals who have a need to know.

When a nurse is asked about a patient's health, she should reply that she cannot disclose any personal medical information. She could suggest that individuals contact the patient directly. She could also inform the patient about the inquiry and clarify who can have information and what information can be shared. The patient's instructions should be documented, to establish that the patient's right to confidentiality has been observed.

Case 31

I have found that patients who are terminally ill often don't want their families to know how close to death they are because they don't want them to be depressed. A patient with bowel cancer that had metastasized told me: "I know I'm dying, but I don't want them to know." He wants to pretend that he is getting better. I disagree. I think his family should know he is dying. **Should I tell his family the truth?**

Case 31 raises the important question of whether families have the right to be informed that a patient is terminally ill, even if the patient wishes to keep this information from them. Based on their rights to self-determination, competent patients have the moral right to determine what medical information about them is confidential, to decide who is to have access to details about their health, and to control the extent of any individual's access to that information. This includes deciding which family members, if any, are informed about the patient's medical condition. If they wish, patients can designate someone other than a family member, such as a life partner or a close friend, as a person who should have access to all patient information. Families do not generally have the right to choose what information they will have or who should be told the patient's diagnosis or prognosis. Patients can indeed refuse permission for any such discussions with their families or anyone else.

The patient's ethical right to confidentiality is afforded legal status in federal regulations and state statutes. The Health Insurance Portability and Accountability Act of 1996 (HIPAA) requires permission from a patient to disclose information to anyone except for healthcare professionals involved in the patient's care, for the purpose of health care operations, for the purpose of receiving payment, and "for the public good." In order to ensure that the patient's legal and moral rights are protected, nurses should ask specific questions in their initial assessment to determine what information the patient wishes to keep confidential and who the patient wishes to have access to personal medical information. Nurses should also discuss with the patient the issue of maintaining the confidentiality of any medical record that remains in the home and their concerns about protecting the patient's privacy.

Accordingly, in Case 31, the nurse cannot reveal the patient's terminal prognosis to his family without his permission. However, given that the patient would presumably benefit if they knew he was dying, the nurse should encourage him to reconsider this. The family, too, might benefit from the opportunity to prepare for his impending death.

Though the nurse cannot reveal the prognosis or any confidential information, she nevertheless should not deceive the family herself by providing false information. She could suggest that family members discuss any concerns they have with the patient, if they press her for answers to their questions.

There are some instances where freer access to patient information would be desirable but is prevented or unnecessarily complicated by HIPAA rules. Nurses may believe that HIPAA rules sometimes preclude doing what is best for the patient by preventing them from contacting family or friends to inform them that a home health care patient needs their help. In cases where patients are no longer competent, HIPAA regulations may also complicate the sharing of information with those who are surrogate decision makers for the patient. For example, if a patient has named someone as a health care agent through the process establishing a durable power of attorney for health care, that individual has a legal right to all information necessary to make decisions on behalf of the patient. An ethical issue would arise, nonetheless, if there were personal medical information of a very sensitive nature that the patient had previously required be kept confidential from everyone except health care professionals involved in his care. In such circumstances nurses and other health care professionals should release the minimum information necessary to make reasonable decisions, but attempt to shield sensitive information from disclosure to the extent possible, in order to abide by the previously expressed wishes of the patient.

BREACHING CONFIDENTIALITY

Case 32

Recently, an elderly patient fell and broke her hip. I'm seeing her to help with pain management. Her daughter took her in after she broke her hip. She works, so the patient is home alone during the day. This week she almost fell again. I'm concerned that she is not safe by herself, but she doesn't want me to discuss this with her daughter. She said she doesn't want to upset her. **Should I tell her daughter what happened?**

This patient would ordinarily have the right to require the nurse to keep any personal medical information confidential from her daughter. However, the patient's right to confidentiality is not absolute and may be overridden by the state's duty to protect public health and maintain the integrity of the medical profession. From a legal perspective, the only exceptions to the requirement to maintain the confidentiality of medical information are in cases where disclosure is required or authorized by the law. Legally required disclosures of otherwise confidential information fall into three categories: (1) disclosures required by subpoena; (2) those required by statute to protect public health and welfare such as mandates to report births and deaths, communicable diseases, victims of violent assault, or child abuse and neglect; and (3) disclosure necessary to protect the patient or innocent third party from serious and imminent harm.

Although the courts have affirmed the right to disclose confidential medical information in these sets of circumstances, four limitations regulating the release of confidential information have been outlined. Confidential information must be disclosed in good faith and reasonable care should be given to guarantee that it is accurate, reported fairly, limited to what is necessary for the sake of protection, and given only to the people who need it for the purpose of protection.

In deciding cases based on breaches of confidentiality, the courts consider whether the disclosure was malicious or made in good faith. Breaches of confidentiality deemed malicious could result in the revocation of one's license, being forced to pay punitive damages, and in some states criminal prosecution. Health care providers who breach patient confidentiality are at risk of liability for damages related to invasion of privacy, malpractice, intentional infliction of emotional distress, breach of applicable state confidentiality statutes, and breach of contract. Disclosures of confidential information made in good faith usually involve paying compensatory damages alone.

In situations where the question is whether to reveal confidential information for the benefit of the patient, the best solution is to persuade patients to reveal the information themselves. Although the patient in Case 32 has thus far refused to do this, it is important to explore her reasons for attempting to conceal her injury and deceive her daughter about the risks of staying home alone. She may be afraid of her daughter's reaction when she learns she has nearly fallen again or worried that she will no longer be able to live with her daughter. Whether or not the nurse decides that this situation justifies breaching her patient's confidentiality, she should be sensitive to the consequences her actions will have for the patient's relationship to her daughter and attempt to minimize any adverse results.

Case 33

I have one patient, a twenty-seven-year-old physician with AIDS, who has . moved back home so his parents can take care of him. He has had multiple opportunistic infections and now has nosebleeds all the time, but he refuses to tell them he has AIDS. As a physician, he is well aware of the risks involved in caring for him, so he has decided to tell his parents he has hepatitis because the precautions they have to take are the same. **Don't they have a right to know they're dealing with AIDS?**

This patient's reluctance to reveal the true nature of his illness is understandable, given the stigma that AIDS patients confront and his apparent desire to keep sensitive information about his personal life confidential. However, his parents face substantial risks to their own health if, for example, they are exposed to his blood. This patient's solution is to deceive his parents in a way that he expects will protect them. Since both hepatitis and AIDS require universal precautions, his parents will be advised to take the same precautionary measures they would take if they were dealing with AIDS. For this solution to succeed, his parents must meticulously follow these precautions and thereby avoid exposure to HIV. Do the risks to his parents justify revealing that he has AIDS?

Courts have permitted medical disclosure to third parties when this disclosure is in their "substantial and valid" interest, though different jurisdictions have come to a variety of conclusions regarding the duty health care professionals have to protect third parties from HIV transmission. For example, the Alaska Supreme Court found that a doctor could reveal his patient's HIV status to the patient's wife, against the patient's wishes, without incurring liability. Other jurisdictions have prohibited the disclosure of such information. Though not uniform, current case law reflects the position that where a health care provider knows or should know that the patient's HIV status poses a serious risk to identifiable third parties, there is a duty to warn these third parties.

Risk to others is an important exception to the legal duty to maintain confidentiality, but the risk must be serious, imminent, and likely to be incurred, to justify a breach in confidentiality. There may be no basis for revealing the AIDS diagnosis in this case, because the family has been instructed to follow universal precautions. It is unclear, though, whether they would be more likely to observe these precautions if they knew that they risked exposure to HIV instead of hepatitis.

Any decision to breach confidentiality in Case 32 should weigh the effect on the relationship the patient has to his parents. Disclosure of the AIDS diagnosis, and thereby the revelation that their son has deceived them about something this important, would impact this family relationship in a considerable and perhaps unpredictable way, possibly with significant consequences for the patient. If a nurse or physician decides that this information must be disclosed, the patient first should be given the opportunity to reveal the diagnosis himself, with the clear understanding that confidentiality will be breached if it is necessary to protect his family.

The agency ethics committee could be a good sounding board to discuss this case. It would be helpful to hear how others would weigh the costs and benefits of maintaining confidentiality or, alternatively, revealing the diagnosis against the patient's wishes. Although ethics committees typically do not make binding decisions, open discussion can clarify the issues and help an individual nurse determine what other nurses consider acceptable resolutions to this dilemma.

Case 34

> I have a new patient, an Hispanic man who is a recent immigrant from the Dominican Republic. He has to learn to give himself insulin injections. When I went to his house, I found out that neither he nor his wife can understand English. She got the neighbor to translate. I was explaining diabetes and insulin injections when all of a sudden the family kneeled down and started praying. I have no idea what the neighbor was saying. **How can I make sure that a patient who doesn't speak English gets correct information and still protect his confidentiality?**

When nurses and patients do not speak the same language, nurses are compelled to use other people to impart essential information, as they strive to educate patients about their health and to teach them what they need to know in order to care for themselves. Using others to disclose medical information to patients raises issues about confidentiality, as well as issues about truthful and full disclosure of the information required for informed consent. The rights of patients can best be protected if a professional interpreter is available to accompany a nurse to a patient's home. Still, coordinating schedules with interpreters and finding appropriate materials in the patient's language can be difficult, with the result that a nurse could arrive at a home without the ideal resources to address the needs of the patient. Sometimes, as in this case, the language problems are not fully apparent until the initial home visit.

In the absence of a professional interpreter, or the unavailability of telephone translation services, it seems natural to turn to neighbors or family members, even children, who speak English to provide the necessary translations. Yet, this solution may compromise informed consent. Family members often are unreliable translators, for they sometimes downplay bad news or are unable to accurately communicate medical information.

Patients relinquish some of their privacy, too, when a family member or neighbors are used as translators. What is most troubling is that they forfeit the opportunity to keep information confidential prior to knowing what will be revealed. This is particularly problematic when children are used to translate. Because it is the patient's right to decide whether medical information should be revealed to someone else, the nurse in this case should warn the patient that information will be disclosed that he may not want others to know. She could then make it clear that the patient can stop the discussion at any point if he should decide that he no longer wishes the details of his medical condition revealed in this way, and they can resume their discussion when a professional interpreter is available. That may be inconvenient, but such steps should be taken if necessary to avoid revealing medical information the patient wants to keep confidential.

CONFIDENTIAL INFORMATION AND SUICIDE

Case 35

I'm very upset about one of my patients who died recently, a young man with testicular cancer who was living with his parents. He sent me e-mail almost every day. Sometimes he just had questions about his health, but other times he shared very personal thoughts. We talked a lot about death. About a month ago, I suspected that he was considering suicide, so I had a social worker talk to him. After that he seemed less anxious and he became peaceful. His condition appeared to stabilize, so I was surprised when he died last Friday. The next day I found a suicide note in my e-mail from him. I know no one suspects this. **Should I tell anyone what I know?**

Ethically, the nurse may have the obligation to maintain the confidentiality of this information. Apparently the patient expected this to remain confidential, because he only revealed the truth in a private message to the nurse. It seems reasonable to conclude that he did not want his family to know he committed suicide, given that he did not leave a suicide note for them to find. In the absence of any overt medical evidence indicating suicide, it would be easy for the nurse to keep this secret.

From a legal perspective, however, there is an obligation to produce evidence of the mode of death of an individual. Failure to do so could be regarded as an obstruction of justice. This is a situation where law and morality seem to conflict. The nurse is legally bound to report that she suspects suicide to the physician, though she may be morally bound by confidentiality to avoid disclosing directly to the family what her patient wanted to be kept a secret. If she does reveal what she knows to the authorities, she will probably be unable to prevent the family from eventually finding out that their son committed suicide. There is no easy resolution to the dilemma in this situation.

Case 36

I have a patient who has end-stage cirrhosis. He lives with his son. Yesterday he said to me, "I think I'll shoot myself." He has just decided that he's had enough. I know he hasn't told anyone else this. I tried to warn his son. "He's dying. You don't know what he might do." **Should I say anything else?**

Although nurses have the obligation to keep information from and about patients confidential, another legal exception to the duty to maintain confidentiality exists when patients threaten suicide, as in Case 36. The nurse must inform the patient that, both legally and professionally, she is required to report a patient's threats of suicide to the physician. The physician must then make a decision regarding detention and civil commitment based on the likelihood of imminent harm to self. Physicians are responsible for knowing and abiding by the procedures governing civil commitment, but it is unlikely that this patient would be considered mentally ill and subject to involuntary commitment for his remarks.

Many health care professionals, including nurses, are convinced that it is possible for a patient to make a rational decision that the burdens of continued existence outweigh the benefits. Others take the position that anyone who threatens or attempts suicide is necessarily depressed or mentally incompetent, thus denying the possibility of a rational suicide. According to this view, paternalistic intervention is always warranted. On the whole, contemporary law reflects the position that the duty to prevent suicide generally overrides a patient's right to make such a decision, even if it is considered rational.

Though there is a legal justification for breaching confidentiality and revealing the patient's suicidal comments to his physician, there is still the moral question of what the nurse would be justified in saying to the patient's son. Under normal circumstances, the patient has the right to expect personal conversations with his nurse to be kept confidential. Revealing this information to his son would be a breach of confidentiality that would only be morally justified if it was necessary to protect the patient. Certainly nurses should act to safeguard patients, but that may be possible to do in this case without disclosing this suicidal conversation to the patient's son.

The nurse should respond to this conversation by taking steps to protect the patient. She can use his comment as an opportunity for a discussion of his fears and concerns, and, if she is able to determine the basis for the patient's significant dissatisfaction with his life, she can advocate for any treatment he needs for pain, depression, or anxiety. Another option is to recommend that he talk with a social worker or clergy. Finally, the nurse should discuss with the patient the effect his suicide would have on his family. Presumably, he would want to spare them any unnecessary unhappiness and perhaps he has not thought carefully about these consequences.

PROTECTING A PATIENT'S PRIVACY

Case 37

One of my patients is a Cambodian man who is on service for wound care. There are always a lot of people there when I arrive and they remain throughout the dressing changes. This is apparently what is expected in his culture. I sense that the patient is very uncomfortable with this because he has no privacy at all, but he won't say anything to them. **Should I do something to protect his privacy when he allows them to stay?**

The issue in Case 37 is how a nurse should respond when a patient acquiesces in violations of a fundamental right such as privacy, given the nurse's professional obligation to protect patient rights. The right to privacy is based on the right to self-determination: competent patients have the right to determine who should have access to their private sphere. Nurses can protect patients from unwanted intrusions upon privacy by affording them the opportunity to decide who is to have access to their bodies, to the extent that it is feasible. Thus, under ordinary circumstances, nurses should accept their patients' decisions concerning who should be present when caring for them.

The idea that an individual should be afforded privacy for treatment is often an alien idea in cultures that have strong social communities. In these communities, an individual is expected to welcome the constant presence of others throughout an illness and recuperation. These cultural practices engender expectations that can complicate a nurse's attempts to preserve patients' privacy. Patients from such cultures may, in fact, waive their right to private treatment. Nurses must respect this choice and support the presence of others when this is desired.

In Case 37, however, the patient's apparent uncomfortableness indicates that he may wish more privacy than is customary in his cultural tradition. The nurse should attempt to provide the patient an opportunity to express his thoughts about this and she should make it clear that the decision to allow any one else to be there is his decision alone. These efforts must be undertaken with sensitivity to the significance of the expectations and practices of his culture and the possible consequences any privacy restrictions he imposes may have for his relationships to the members of his group.

Case 38

I'm taking care of a thirteen-year-old girl who was in a bad car accident. She may not be able to walk normally again. I'm sure she is frightened by this possibility, but I can't talk with her about her injury or her fears because one of her parents is always there. They won't allow her to discuss it. **Should I ask them to leave us alone?**

Teenagers, though not legally adults, are old enough to deserve some privacy when they are patients. Thus, nurses should respect their physical privacy to the greatest extent possible, as well as allow them an opportunity for private discussions about their health concerns. By assessing an individual teenage patient's maturity, nurses can determine what limits to medical privacy are appropriate to impose in a particular case.

Because they refuse to allow their daughter the opportunity to talk privately with the nurse, these parents are in fact interfering in the nurse-patient relationship. The nurse should explain the value of establishing a professional relationship with their daughter and encourage the parents to support this by respecting their daughter's privacy. Parents sometimes need to be educated about the issue of privacy and the psychological needs of a teenager who faces illness or disability

More importantly, this teenager should be able to discuss her prognosis and concerns and assent to any decisions made about her care. Her parents are effectively preventing her involvement in those matters. The nurse should support the daughter's participation in medical decisions affecting her. If necessary, the nurse can offer to contact a social worker who can help the family address these issues.

PROTECTING FAMILY PRIVACY

Case 39

I see myself as an invited guest in a patient's home. Sometimes I'm a witness to private family matters, so I am very careful about what I document. As an example, I have one situation where the patient's son is bizarre. He's taking good care of her, but he is definitely strange. When I was early for my appointment last week, he answered the door in his mother's dress. She told me he has always worn her clothes around the house and she asked me not to document this. **Should I keep this family secret?**

Some family secrets such as this may be revealed inadvertently when nurses visit a patient's home, and, understandably, families expect their secrets to remain private. A family waives its claim to family privacy to some extent, however, when home health care is provided. Nurses are required to record detailed background information about a patient's home and family life, such as information about living arrangements and safety hazards in the home. When further information about a patient's family life comes to the attention of home health care nurses, the ethical question is the extent of a family's right to privacy and confidentiality in these circumstances.

There is some family information that appears to have no bearing on the health and safety of the patient and may pose a risk to someone's reputation and employment if it is revealed. If a patient's primary caregiver is a homosexual partner, for example, that information may be sensitive. Given that family information is justifiably documented as part of an assessment of a patient's risks in being treated at home, information that is relevant to the health, safety or well-being of the patient should be recorded. Other information should be protected. Accordingly, in Case 39, the written record should include mention of the son as the family caregiver and should document the extent and quality of the care he provides for his mother. Other observations about his behavior should not be part of the written record unless it is relevant to his mother's well-being.

Given their access to very personal information, home health care nurses should be sensitive to privacy and confidentiality concerns and pay careful attention to the issue of what to document. The burgeoning use of computerized records and the oversight increasingly exercised by health care insurers exacerbate these issues about protecting the confidentiality of information and respecting patient and family privacy. In general, confidentiality and privacy should be protected to the greatest degree possible that is compatible with the safety and well-being of patients and others.

ANALYSIS OF CASE 29

Case 29 describes the situation of an HIV patient who needs medications he cannot afford. He refuses to let the nurse contact his parents for help because he has not told them he is HIV positive. The ethical issue is whether the nurse should disclose his medical needs so that he can get his medications.

Undoubtedly, this patient would benefit if he could get the necessary medications. A nurse focused on promoting his health and addressing his pain may believe that this would ethically justify contacting his parents to disclose that he needs their help. Similarly, nurses caring for elderly patients may wish to contact their adult children to inform them that they must step in to help a parent who can no longer cope. Nurses' obligations to protect patient health and safety support these disclosures, but at the same time, these actions would conflict with fundamental patient rights to confidentiality and the nurses' duty to respect patient rights.

The basis for the moral and legal requirement of confidentiality of personal medical information is the right of self-determination. Competent patients have the right to determine who has access to medical information and to decide the extent to which information can be revealed to others. From a legal perspective, confidentiality can only be breached when the law requires or authorizes disclosure of information. Disclosure is required in three situations: a subpoena has been issued for the information; disclosure is necessary to protect public health and welfare; and, disclosure is necessary to protect the patient or an innocent third party from serious and imminent harm. In all other cases, the patient must specifically give consent to have information shared.

The consequences, therefore, cannot justify disclosing information about a patient, except in the three kinds of situations identified above. Though the patient's parents would presumably want to help him obtain the medications he cannot afford, and the patient would thus clearly benefit in that way, the nurse should not decide to breach confidentiality on the basis of those benefits. The rules about confidentiality are not based on consequences, but on the right of an individual to have control over information about him or herself.

Moreover, given the significance family relationships have for the individual's life, the patient himself should be able to determine what his parents know about his illness. He can then satisfy the responsibility to show care for his parents in the way that he wishes, and he may minimize the harm to his family. The nurse could attempt to persuade the patient to reveal the nature of his illness to his parents, or she could seek other resources to help him pay for his medications, but that is as much as she can ethically do.

ETHICAL CRITERIA

- The patient has the right to confidentiality, which includes the right to determine whether to disclose confidential information to anyone.
- The patient has a right to privacy.

PRACTICAL STRATEGIES

When others ask questions:

- Reply that the patient's health cannot be discussed.
- Report others' inquiries to the patient.

When revealing confidential information to others could benefit the patient:

- Encourage the patient to reveal this information.
- Secure the patient's permission to arrange a family conference.
- Understand the legal exceptions to confidentiality.

When revealing confidential information could prevent harm to others:

- Encourage the patient to reveal the information to those at risk.
- Determine whether the risk of harm is serious, imminent, and unavoidable, and, if so, report to the agency supervisor.
- Consult the agency supervisor and the ethics committee for advice in cases of uncertainty.

When interpreters are necessary:

- Try to obtain the patient's permission when an unofficial interpreter is used.
- Protect confidentiality by revealing no more information than is necessary.

When patients commit suicide:

- Determine what the law requires.
- Maintain confidentiality as far as possible.

When patients threaten suicide:

- Discuss with the patient the impact that the decision would have on the family.
- Seek professional mental health services for the patient.
- Inform the patient about the legal limits to confidentiality.

When the patient's privacy is compromised by the presence of others:

- Let the patient decide what is acceptable.
- Protect the patient against privacy violations.
- Discuss privacy rights with the family.

When the family's privacy is at stake:

- Be sensitive to family concerns about revealing embarrassing information.
- Document only what is necessary to ensure the patient's safety and the safety of others.

Chapter 5

PATIENTS WHO DO NOT
"FOLLOW ORDERS"

Patients and families sometimes fail to follow physicians' "orders," despite the fact that the patient's health appears to depend on their compliance with the plan of care. This nonadherence frustrates nurses' attempts to meet the ethical responsibility to protect and promote the health of patients.

Case 40

One of my cases involves a patient who has intractable pain, congestive heart failure, hypertension and an anxiety disorder. Her husband says, "Whatever she wants, I do. If she wants to go to the ER, I take her." Last week they went to the Emergency Room three times, Thursday, Saturday, and Monday. If she doesn't like one ER, they stop at another ER on the way home. Sometimes it's for pain, sometimes it's diarrhea, sometimes it's constipation. She has medications she doesn't want to take, so they play around with her medications and then run to the ER when a problem develops. It's very frustrating because they're not managing her pain and they're jeopardizing her health. **What should I do?**

General Issues

- **What actions are justified when a patient does not "follow orders"?**
- **What should nurses do when family caregivers do not follow the plan of care?**
- **When is a nurse justified in refusing to care for a patient who does not "follow orders"?**

66

INTRODUCTION

The process of informed consent requires health care professionals to ask competent individuals to accept or reject the medical treatments that are recommended by their physicians. Individuals thereby have the ultimate responsibility for decisions about their treatment and their own health. This responsibility, together with the rise of health care consumerism and the availability of Internet web sites as a source of medical information, encourages people to educate themselves about their health problems and the alternatives for treatment. Increasingly, individuals are led to scrutinize the recommendations of health care professionals before making important medical decisions and to question the health advice and the authority of physicians and nurses.

In hospitals, however, the longstanding tradition of unquestioning obedience to medical authority still generally prevails. Though hospitalized patients can exercise their rights to refuse medication or treatments, they usually consent and are prepared to follow the doctor's orders. People are understandably motivated to adhere closely to a recommended plan of care when they have an illness or condition serious enough to require hospitalization. Moreover, once they have consented, hospitalized patients seldom have the opportunity to neglect treatment, even if they are not motivated to "follow orders" conscientiously.

When patients leave the authoritarian hospital atmosphere for the sanctity of their own homes, family caregivers or patients themselves are expected to take over the responsibility for a patient's health care. Assigned this responsibility, patients and families may question the advice they have received for the patient's care and take it upon themselves to determine a plan of care. Family caregivers may question the necessity for a treatment, for example, and decide to disregard that part of the patient's care. Further, family caregivers can become negligent and nonadherent when providing care is inconvenient, unpleasant, or burdensome for them. Once home, patients who do not want to follow a doctor's orders can find it easy to postpone or skip a treatment, or to stop taking a medication altogether.

If patients have consented to treatment but then do not follow through, their actual wishes are unclear. Nurses must contend with the ethical complexity of distinguishing what is in reality a treatment refusal, from a situation where a patient is not following through with treatment because of problems with side effects, for example. They also often face the professional and ethical challenge of caring for patients who thwart their best efforts to promote their health.

WHEN PATIENTS DO NOT "FOLLOW ORDERS"

Case 41

> This patient lives in a rat-infested tenement, with trash, spoiled food, and even dog feces scattered around. She is an insulin-dependent diabetic who is totally nonadherent with her diet and refuses any suggestions I make for her care. Yesterday, I was so concerned about her cellulitis that I sent her to the ER for treatment. She walked out of the ER because she didn't want to be admitted to the hospital. She wanted to be home to take care of her grandson. **What should I do when a patient doesn't seem to value her health enough to follow recommendations for treatment she clearly needs?**

Patients who reject advice designed to protect them from serious health risks are difficult patients to care for, because they do not appear to share the nurse's fundamental commitment to their health. For the nurse's efforts to promote their health to be successful, patients must comply with the behaviors and treatments that will serve that goal. Most people will cooperate with healthcare professionals and follow their treatment plans conscientiously, because they value their own health more than anything else. They want to live as long as they can, with the highest quality of life, and they are willing to do whatever it takes to accomplish that. Others, however, sacrifice or compromise their own health and well-being for the sake of something they value more highly. Some pregnant women may refuse chemotherapy drugs in order to protect a fetus, professionals sometimes neglect their own health to pursue a career goal, others drive themselves too hard in order to earn a living to support a family—all of these people challenge the assumption that good health will always be the highest value for patients.

Patients' relationships and their family obligations certainly may be more important to patients than their own health. To respect patients' own values, nurses should encourage them to "follow orders" to the greatest extent that is compatible with the values and commitments that are important to them. This could require some creative suggestions to accommodate a patient's family responsibilities and thus to facilitate a patient's adherence to a plan of care. From an ethical perspective, nurses can educate, urge, and cajole in order to get a patient to follow the plan, but when the decisions patients make to reject recommendations about their health are informed and voluntary, this is as far as nurses can go to promote adherence.

A difficulty in some cases is determining whether a patient's failure to follow health advice actually constitutes self-neglect. This patient's living conditions, her failure to take care of herself, and her refusal to adhere to a plan to address her diabetes raise the possibility of self-neglect. She has also significantly jeopardized her health by refusing emergency treatment for a serious medical problem. Though she apparently regards her family responsibilities as more important than her own health problems, a choice that others might also make, her ongoing failure to protect her health may constitute self-neglect. When a patient's nonadherence plainly constitutes self-neglect, questions about the patient's competence also arise. The nurse should inform the patient's physician and her supervisor of her concerns.

Case 42

My patient is HIV-positive, but he's still drinking and using drugs, and he is not taking his medications. It's a horrible medication regimen and the medications have really awful side effects. This is very upsetting for me because he's just not following the plan at all. Now he has pneumonia. **How far should I go to provide care for a patient who apparently isn't making any effort to improve his own health?**

Patients who refuse to follow any health advice and persist in self-destructive behavior thwart the conscientious efforts of nurses to fulfill their professional and moral responsibilities. An important part of nursing responsibilities is to establish a caring relationship, with the patient's participation in planning care, which may seem almost impossible when patients resist and are significantly nonadherent. The situation with this patient illustrates the resulting frustration and ethical difficulty nurses face when their efforts to care for a patient appear to be futile.

An important response to a patient's nonadherent behavior is to explore the reasons the patient is not following the plan of care. If the patient disagrees with the goals of treatment, finds the side effects of medications intolerable, or is unable to fit the requirements of the care plan into the daily schedule of the family, nurses can involve the patient in the quest for adaptations that will facilitate adherence. As an example, this patient's physician may be able to recommend a medication regimen that the patient could follow with less difficulty. Additional concerns about the patient's drug and alcohol addictions and his mental health also need to be addressed, though the patient may refuse to seek treatment for those problems, which is his right as a competent patient.

Once the nurse has assessed the possible causes of a patient's nonaderence, addressed them to the best of her ability, and informed the patient's physician, she has done as much as she can ethically do. If the patient's behavior continues to impede the nurse's efforts to provide professional nursing care, she is justified in asking to have another nurse assigned to the case. From an ethical perspective, no one is required to persist in what are futile efforts to provide care.

Case 43

My patient had a heart attack at the age of forty-four. She's taking several heart medications. Now she has stomach problems, so she thinks she's toxic from the digitalis and she has stopped taking it. She's done a lot of searching for information on the Internet, talking to some doctor in California about natural treatments for heart disease. My concern is that she may be neglecting the standard care for her heart condition, but she says she just wants to take charge of her own treatment. **What is my responsibility if a patient is 'playing doctor'?**

It appears that this patient may trust her own ideas about her illness and treatments more than the experienced judgments of doctors and nurses. Some patients do try to become their own "doctors," attempting to diagnose their illnesses and prescribe treatments for themselves, and implicitly rejecting the value of medical expertise. When patients risk their health by refusing medications or using alternative treatments that may be dangerous or may interfere with the standard medical treatments, nurses are justified in taking an aggressive stance in expressing their misgivings about the patients' choices. Most importantly, a patient who reaches her own conclusions about a symptom and then stops a medication, must be informed of the risks of rejecting standard medical treatments for a serious condition, and her physician must be informed. Nevertheless, patients have the responsibility for their own health care choices, and they can reject nursing and medical judgment if they wish.

Patients can also reject the advice of any physician and seek a second opinion from another. The problem here is that the second opinion is from a doctor whose qualifications are unknown and whose only contact with the patient is through the Internet. An added concern is that the patient is translating this information into treatment recommendations for her own care. Though the easy availability of Internet resources encourages patients to educate themselves about diseases, treatments, and medicines, which is basically good, such information should be subjected to a critical appraisal and should not be the basis for rejecting standard care without careful consideration. For that reason, the patient should be encouraged to initiate a discussion with her physician about the information and treatments she has discovered on the Internet.

Case 44

I have a patient in his eighties who lives alone. He is a very frail man, weighing only about ninety pounds. I see him to check his blood pressure. His doctor put him on a new medication, but he's not taking any of his medications. He told me he just made his funeral arrangements. I'm wondering whether he has stopped his medications because he wants to die. **What should I do if he continues to refuse his medications?**

Because patients who refuse a medication may have developed unexpected symptoms or may find a treatment regimen too difficult to follow, the first step is to assess the reasons for the patient's nonadherence. In some cases, patients who are nonadherent may be depressed and may conclude that it is not worth continuing treatment. Accordingly, this patient should be screened for depression and, if necessary, treatment for mental health problems should be recommended. He can, of course, reject that recommendation.

Competent patients have the right to reject any recommended treatment, even if that will result in death. A patient who wishes to stop treatment could choose to do so, without discussing it with health care professionals or anyone else, by simply refusing to follow the doctor's orders. Thus, if patients do not comply with medical recommendations and have not identified any reasons for their nonadherence, nurses should act to ensure that they are not depressed, that they intend to stop treatment, and that they fully understand the consequences of their nonadherence. It is important that these patients be offered any other treatments their conditions warrant and continue to have access to nursing care if they should decide to accept it. In this case, that is especially important, because there are medications that would enhance the comfort of a dying patient. This patient might wish to accept those comfort measures, even though he is refusing other medications. Finally, nurses must always notify the physician of any significant changes in a patient's condition and inform physicians when patients are nonadherent.

Case 45

I have a patient with a skin disorder who was put on an antianxiety pill for treatment. After her husband died recently, she stopped taking her medication. She developed the skin problem again but she won't take the anti-anxiety pill. **How should I respond when a mental health patient will not follow the recommended treatment?**

The challenge often presented when a patient is nonadherent is to distinguish what is actually a competent treatment refusal from situations where the patient fails to understand the reason for the treatment, finds the medication or treatment too difficult to endure, or is seriously neglecting her own health. In this case, there appears to be no evidence of self-neglect, thus the nurse should focus on educating the patient further about the reason for the medication and attempt to determine whether there is a side effect or some other reason that the patient has rejected this medication. Because competent patients being treated for mental illness have the same right to refuse treatment that all competent patients have, there is little else than a nurse can do ethically.

Case 46

I have a Southeast Asian patient who was referred by the TB clinic. He has tuberculosis and diabetes. It's hard to convince him that he needs medications. We're in there daily, testing his blood sugar, making sure he takes his TB medications and his insulin. **How can I meet my responsibilities to care for a patient who rejects Western ideas about health?**

Patients may value their own health highly, but reject the standard Western ideas and practices designed to promote health. If patients do not accept the idea that what is recommended will actually help them regain their health, it is difficult to persuade them to "follow orders" and to allow appropriate nursing interventions.

Where cultural differences exist, nurses should first of all act to ensure that patients are fully informed about their illnesses and the consequences of nonadherence. Because this patient could be relatively new to Western culture and medicine and perhaps has language difficulties as well, this may best be accomplished through the use of an appropriate interpreter or the cooperation of a health clinic allied with the local southeast Asian population. The recommendations of physicians and nurses and, more importantly, the reasons for accepting Western medicine, must be made as clear as possible to the patient. If the patient still wishes to make an informed, voluntary decision to reject treatment, that decision should be respected.

As long as the well-being of other people is not at risk, the patient has the right to reject what Western medicine has to offer, no matter what the consequences are for his own health. However, if he has active tuberculosis, he must follow the treatment regimen to protect others from contracting the disease. Consequently, the appropriate public health authorities will have to become involved in that case if he continues to resist the recommendations for treatment.

WHEN FAMILY CAREGIVERS DO NOT FOLLOW THE PLAN OF CARE

Case 47

My patient is an infant. At birth, the baby had multiple life-threatening conditions and extensive brain damage, but her teenage mother wanted the doctors to do everything they could to save her. Now the girl and her mother are trying to care for this baby at home, and they are overwhelmed. I'm sure the baby is not getting all the treatments and feedings she needs. Still, if I try to get them outside help, they could be judged guilty of neglect and lose the baby. **What's the right thing to do in a case like this?**

When families do not provide the care they are expected to give, the first step is to inquire about the reasons for their nonadherence.

Most families sincerely want to provide good care, but some care-givers may be limited in their ability to understand the requirements of the plan of care or they may have difficulty learning the skills that are needed. Nurses can then offer further education and skills training or, if possible, adapt a plan of care to their capabilities.

Unfortunately, it may be necessary to remove a patient from home health care if family caregivers consistently fail to provide the required care. Even then, competent patients could decide that they wish to remain at home, with family taking the responsibility for their care, despite these deficiencies. However, if the patient is an infant or an incompetent adult, individuals who lack the capacity to make that decision for themselves, the best interest of the patient should determine whether the individual remains in home health care.

The best interest of the patient can generally be determined by evaluating the consequences of the alternative settings for providing patient care. For example, is it better for this infant to stay at home, even with compromised care, than to be removed from home health care? Her mother and grandmother are striving to provide what she needs, and the benefits of living in a loving home are significant. However, the infant will not thrive if she does not receive adequate nutrition or necessary treatments. The costs and benefits of compromised care must be weighed against the costs to the infant and the family if the child is removed from the home.

Yet, when the level of care the mother and grandmother are able to provide is so poor that it is precipitating an immediate threat to the infant's life, or constitutes abuse or neglect, the infant should be removed from the home. Given the seriousness of this possibility, the nurse needs more information about the level of care actually being provided by the infant's family before proceeding. If she concludes that the infant is receiving inadequate care, she must report that, even though the consequence is that the mother may lose custody of her infant.

Case 48

I have a dying patient who was always the controller in the family. Now that he cannot take care of himself, his wife is in control. The power in the family has reversed. He complains to me that he is experiencing a lot of pain. I suspect his wife is not giving him the pain medications as often as he needs them.

His daughter told me she thinks her mother is getting her revenge. **What should I do?**

The wife's reasons for apparently withholding pain medications are unknown. Well-meaning families may stop following a plan of care for various reasons. Families focused on keeping a patient happy may resist imposing treatments that are painful or unpleasant in any way, and they may allow patients to enjoy old habits that a physician has now forbidden. Others who want the patient to make his own decisions will not impose treatment if a patient objects, because they want the patient to have the dignity of controlling his own treatment. In other situations, families may be physically or psychologically unable to make the patient comply. For example, children or spouses who are used to accepting the authority of a patient may find it difficult to insist on the prescribed treatment when a patient is uncooperative. Finally, families that are overwhelmed by the role of caregiver may forget or neglect certain aspects of care. The appropriate response in all of these cases is to renew efforts to teach the family about the need for the recommended treatment and to arrange a family discussion to address the difficulties the family has in providing care.

On the other hand, families who are actually hostile to the patient they are supposed to care for may not be sufficiently motivated to follow treatment plans conscientiously. Nurses can address this hostility through their efforts to educate a family about the patient's illness and the effect it will have on the patient's behavior. Families will perhaps be less hostile if they fully understand the consequences of the illness and the effects of their nonadherence. A discussion with the patient's wife to clarify the use of pain medications could itself solve the problem in this particular case. In addition, there may be other ways to succeed in getting the patient the care he needs. There could be other methods for delivering the pain medication, such as a morphine patch or a longer-acting pain medication, that would not rely as much on his wife's cooperation. If a patient is in imminent danger because of neglect or abuse, then of course a nurse should report the situation to her supervisor and the appropriate authorities.

REFUSING TO CARE FOR A PATIENT WHO DOES NOT "FOLLOW ORDERS"

Case 49

I have a patient who has loads of medical problems. The real problem, though, is that she is uncooperative, irritable, and suspicious, and she never has a kind word for anyone. I try not to have other nurses cover for me, because every nurse who has been there came back with a horror story. I seem to be the only nurse she likes. Now she needs a colonoscopy. Her doctor wants to do this on an outpatient basis but she wants to stay overnight in the hospital. Yesterday her blood pressure shot up. I think she skipped her medicine because she thought she would have to be hospitalized. **What should I do when a patient tries to manipulate the system in order to get unnecessary treatment?**

This patient's nonadherent behavior is apparently intended to force the physician to meet her demands for hospitalization, which is not necessary for the procedure she needs. The subsequent legal and ethical issue is whether the patient's manipulative, nonadherent behavior warrants the termination of services by the agency. Home health care agencies normally inform patients of their rights and responsibilities, in writing, when they are admitted. One of the responsibilities that is identified is the patient's responsibility to follow the plan of care established by the physician and to comply with the instructions of other health care professionals which are intended to accomplish the doctor's orders. A patient's nonadherence, or the failure of family caregivers to follow a physician's orders, could thus justify withdrawing services, on the grounds that the patient or the family has not fulfilled these responsibilities.

To terminate services, the agency, the physician, or other professional caregiver is required to notify the patient in writing, giving an explanation for the withdrawal. The caregiver must recommend continued treatment if necessary, provide a reasonable amount of time for an effective termination date, and offer to make the patient's medical records available to the new agency and physician, with the patient's consent. Failure to meet these terms could result in charges of patient abandonment, resulting in tort liability.

If the agency does not move to terminate services, the patient's behavior might justify a request by the nurse to withdraw from the case, on the grounds that this patient's nonadherent behavior fails to satisfy her responsibilities as a patient. Nonetheless, given her success in establishing a relationship where others have failed, she may decide to continue as this patient's nurse. She may believe she has an obligation to maintain this relationship, especially if she is convinced the patient is unlikely to establish an adequate caring relationship with a new nurse. The issue is essentially an issue about character. Do her own ethical standards compel her to continue caring for this patient?

Case 50

My patient has chronic disease which is very hard to manage. He's in and out of the hospital. They treat him, send him home, and in a week, he's in trouble again. It's obvious he is not following the plan of care. When he was admitted to the hospital the last time, the agency decided they would not take him back. They were firm. He was calling the agency three or four times a day, yelling and cursing at everyone, and he was not doing what he was supposed to do, so they wouldn't have him back on service. But this time he has heart failure, which qualifies for skilled visits, and the agency has agreed to take him back. We currently have a contract with him that specifies that he will be discharged from service if he does not follow the plan of care. **Does my responsibility to my patient mean that I should ignore his nonadherence so he won't be discharged?**

Nurses have a fundamental responsibility to promote a patient's well-being, which may seem to require that they act to protect a patient's continued access to care, even when the patient is nonadherent. Home health care agencies, though, commonly operate under agreements that specify patient adherence as a requirement for continued care. When patients or family caregivers have been persistently nonadherent, agencies sometimes establish a contract with the provision that services will be withdrawn if the plan of care is not followed, as has been done in Case 50. It is clear that the agency can end the relationship with the patient if he does not satisfy the agreed-upon conditions for providing home health care. Because the nurse is required to keep accurate records, she cannot avoid noting any patient nonadherence that is significant, which may result in his dismissal from services.

An agreement outlining responsibilities and rights, however, does not adequately define the nurse-patient relationship that is the basis for providing nursing care. Most important, a contract specifying the conditions for services does not express the richness of the caring human relationship that often develops between nurse and patient. Conforming strictly to the letter of an agreement may not satisfy a nurse's ethical responsibility to a patient. Nurses who believe that their care is substantially helping patients may feel an obligation to continue in spite of a patient's frequent nonadherence to the treatment plan, which would justify withdrawing services. If a nurse believes that a patient will benefit from remaining on service, she should be the patient's advocate with the agency and argue against dismissal, despite difficult behavior. On the other hand, the nurse also has moral rights of her own to request withdrawal if the patient becomes hostile.

Ultimately, in accepting home health care, patients themselves, directly or through their caregivers, take on responsibility for their continuing care. Though nurses can appropriately attempt to persuade patients to "follow orders," there is a limit to what they can and should do when confronted with an uncooperative patient. Competent patients who do not behave in accordance with treatment plans cannot ethically be manipulated or coerced, given that they have the right to refuse treatment. At the same time, competent patients have no guaranteed right to nursing care if their actions make such care ineffective or inappropriate. Agencies and individual nurses may withdraw, as long as it does not leave a patient totally abandoned and without needed nursing care, that is, they can transfer care to another nurse or agency. The case of incompetent patients is different, for the responsibility for care lies with the caregiver. Nurses have the responsibility of assuring that the patient is receiving adequate care. When education of caregivers and careful monitoring of patient care are not effective and the situation is serious enough, a report of medical neglect or abuse should be made to the appropriate authorities.

Analysis of Case 40

Case 40 involves a patient who is nonadherent with her medications, develops medical problems as a result, and then makes several trips to the emergency room. It is obvious that the patient's nonadherence is jeopardizing her health and well-being. The ethical question is what the nurse should do when a patient does not "follow orders."

The nurse's first response should be to determine whether this is in fact a competent treatment refusal, which is a patient's right. If the patient is exercising her right to refuse treatment, the nurse should respect that decision, under ordinary circumstances. She should ensure that the patient understands the nature of her illnesses and the consequences of nonadherence.

On the other hand, patients may neglect a physician's orders for several reasons: the treatment plan is too difficult to follow, medication side effects are unpleasant, or some other goal or value is more important to the patient than adhering to the plan of care. Nurses should discuss with patients the reasons for nonadherence so that they may address these problems. In each of these cases, nurses may appropriately focus their efforts on acceptable modifications to a plan in response to these concerns, and should discuss with the patient's physician suggestions for changes which require a physician's orders. Accordingly, in Case 40, the nurse should first redouble her efforts to teach the patient and her husband about the effects of their nonadherence on pain management and the patient's quality of life. She should contact the physician and advocate for a change in the medication orders, if she believes that will address the problems the patient and her husband are apparently having with her care.

These responses to nonadherence may not be sufficient in Case 40. With so many visits to the emergency room, something is certainly going wrong. The judgment of both the patient and her husband is questionable, since they are apparently causing her additional health problems by modifying the medication dosages and schedules. The patient's husband appears unwilling to administer medications his wife doesn't want to take and he seems to be reluctant to reject his wife's requests to be taken to the emergency room, perhaps because he does not want to upset her. He may also be overwhelmed by the responsibility of caring for her. The nurse should initiate a discussion with the patient and her husband to inquire about the difficulties they are having with following the patient's plan of care. Once they understand the necessity of following instructions for medications closely, and the consequences of changing dosages and medication schedules, they may "follow orders" more conscientiously. If this fails to address the problems, or if she is concerned about mental illness, self-neglect, or the competence of the family caregiver, she should notify her supervisor and the physician promptly.

In some cases when patients are nonadherent, families and nurses must cope with the frustration of attempting to care for patients who resist their efforts to help them. Based on her rights as a professional nurse, this nurse could request to transfer care to another nurse, in accordance with agency policies and any applicable laws and regulations, if the patient and her husband continue to be nonadherent.

ETHICAL CRITERIA

- A competent patient has the right to refuse to follow the plan of care.
- Nurses have the responsibility to advocate for noncompetent patients whose caregivers fail to follow the plan of care.

PRACTICAL STRATEGIES

When good health is not the patient's highest value:

- Ascertain why the patient is not following the plan of care.
- Educate the patient about the risks involved in nonadherence.
- Be sure that the patient's choice is voluntary.
- Encourage the patient to adhere to the treatment plan as fully as possible.

When a patient's nonadherence endangers someone:

- Explain the risks involved.
- Contact the appropriate authorities to protect innocent third parties, if necessary.

When a patient agrees to treatment but does not follow through:

- Identify the reasons for the patient's behavior.
- Make sure the patient understands the consequences.
- Propose ways to improve adherence.

• Explore modifications in the plan of care that will accommodate patient concerns.

When the patient's family does not follow the plan of care:

• Identify obstacles that interfere with providing care.
• Adapt the plan of care to address the problems.
• Protect the safety of the patient.

When the patient's behavior raises questions about continuation of services:

• Discuss with the patient the reasons for nonadherence and the consequences of the behavior.
• Review with the patient the contract and conditions for continued service.
• Assist the patient with transfer of care if necessary.

Chapter 6

RESPECTING CULTURAL DIFFERENCES

Patients' beliefs about the causes of disease and the treatments that will restore health are shaped by their cultural traditions. These culturally determined beliefs sometimes conflict with the concepts of health and disease that provide the basis for Western nursing practice, a conflict that can be magnified when nursing care is provided in the patient's home.

Case 51

Several Haitian families have recently moved to our community because one of the local churches has agreed to sponsor them. Our agency has been caring for Haitian patients who maintain their cultural practices and accept the traditional ideas about diseases and medicines. Right now, I have a patient who is convinced someone put a curse on her because she suffered complications after she gave birth at home. She isn't taking the medications her physician prescribed because she believes they won't do any good. Instead she's been using a folk remedy. **What should I do about this?**

General Issues

- **How should nurses respond when patients reject Western practices?**
- **When is it acceptable to compromise to accommodate cultural differences?**
- **Are there some cultural practices that should not be tolerated?**

INTRODUCTION

There is a consensus that good nursing care requires what has come to be known as cultural competence. In fact, a requirement for cultural competence has been established in the standards set by the Joint Commission on Accreditation of Healthcare Organizations, which apply to home health care agencies. Achieving cultural competence requires these skills: First, nurses must develop awareness of culturally distinct values and beliefs. This includes becoming aware of the influence of cultural values on nurses' own personal beliefs and behaviors. Second, nurses must foster an attitude of respect for cultural beliefs and an attitude that values cultural differences. Third, nurses must have knowledge of various cultural ideas and practices, especially the beliefs of those populations that they serve. Finally, nurses must develop skills in accommodating cultural differences when providing nursing care.

Recognizing the significance and influence of cultural beliefs must begin with the awareness that cultural ideas and values influence nurses themselves. Most important, there are certain beliefs that function as unstated assumptions underlying Western nursing and medical practices, and these may conflict with the beliefs of people from different cultural backgrounds. One prevalent Western belief is that an important goal of scientific study is to learn about nature in order to control it for human purposes. Research on a condition such as high blood pressure, for example, aims at discovering treatments that will control the natural forces that are responsible for the condition. In contrast, many non-Western cultures seek to understand the natural world in order to be able to work with the elements of nature and to live in harmony with the natural order of things. For those who believe that health results from maintaining the proper harmony or balance of hot and cold elements, for instance, the choice of treatment for high blood pressure depends on whether it will contribute to restoring that balance, rather than its possible use in the defeat of natural forces.

Another characteristic Western belief is that the causes of disease are elements in the physical world such as germs and viruses. Only by responding to these physical causes can medicine eliminate or ameliorate disease and illness. In other cultures, however, the origins of disease may be attributed to forces such as the curse of an enemy or disturbed powers in the spirit world. As a result, Western medicine, which attempts to eliminate the somatic causes, will seem irrelevant or insufficient. If illness is attributed to forces in the spirit world, treating the physical causes of disease will be thought to be ineffective unless a ceremony is held that is designed to make peace with those spiritual forces.

In general, Western cultures expect nurses and physicians to focus primarily on the physical health of patients, to provide effective treatments using drugs or surgical interventions, to act to prolong human life, and to enhance the quality of life by alleviating physical suffering and promoting healthy bodies. Other cultures often place a different value on physical well-being, emphasizing instead the spiritual life of individuals and assigning greater significance to spiritual functioning. Treatments that would jeopardize mental or spiritual awareness, as in the case of a medication that depresses consciousness, may be rejected by some individuals at the end of life in order to maintain the right state of mind. Further, many religious groups place great value on a spiritual life after death. Accordingly, some followers might make medical decisions designed to enhance their spiritual life, even at the expense of their physical well-being.

Explicitly recognizing the beliefs that inform the practice of Western health care fosters an appreciation for the significant differences in the way other individuals and cultures understand the world and their place in it. These cultural differences must be acknowledged by nurses who practice in a hospital setting, but take on an even added significance in the context of the patient's home, where patients' own cultural beliefs dominate. Cultural competence demonstrates respect for patients as individuals with the right to make their own medical decisions and respect for the personal, culturally influenced values which form the basis for their decisions. The ethical challenge for nurses is to satisfy the professional standards of scientific, competent nursing care, while respecting the cultural differences that may lead patients to reject fundamental Western ideals and practices.

WHEN PATIENTS REJECT WESTERN PRACTICES

Case 52

I have a case that involves a patient who suffers from Alzheimer's disease. He is refusing to take the medications his physician prescribed. His family believes that magnets will have an effect, so he is sleeping with magnets under his pillow. He agrees with this idea that the magnets will cure him. **Should I go along with this?**

The important question when patients and their families follow their own cultural practices is whether the practices are seen as harmful in themselves by Western practitioners or appear to be incompatible with a physician's recommended care. Some practices, such as ingesting certain would-be "remedies" in place of medicines known to be effective in treating an illness, are themselves harmful for patients. Other traditional practices are harmful if they prevent, are substituted for, or interfere with the treatment ordered by a physician. Where there is very effective treatment, as with early treatment of breast cancer, time is lost when alternative treatments are tried. Consequently, even if the patient ultimately accepts the recommended therapy, the outcome is likely to be much less favorable.

If the cultural traditions a patient chooses to follow are harmful, nurses have an obligation to act to protect the patient's health. They should expand their efforts to educate patients about their medical condition and the risks involved in any potentially dangerous cultural practices, and must inform a patient's physician when the patient is refusing the recommended treatment. In addition, nurses should attempt to persuade patients to modify cultural practices that are harmful or interfere with effective treatment. Nevertheless, competent patients have the right to reject Western medicine, and that right must be respected.

On the other hand, when cultural practices appear to be harmless and do not compromise the effectiveness of Western medicine, there is no obligation to act to protect patient health or to persuade patients to change these practices.

With respect to the "cure" using magnets, there appears to be no harm in this practice in itself. The harm is done when magnets are substituted for doctor-recommended treatment. If the patient and family can be persuaded to use the magnets in conjunction with the pre-

scribed medications, then the patient has the benefit of Western medicine and the nurse will be demonstrating an attitude of respect for the
family's cultural beliefs. In any case, whether cultural practices are
harmful, incompatible with recommended care, or essentially harmless, nurses must respect patients' cultural beliefs.

Case 53

I have been caring for a number of refugees from Liberia who have their own
ideas about how disease is transmitted. My patient told me that a witch doctor
called her on the phone and issued a curse, and then she became infected with
HIV. I have tried to convince her that she needs to take her medications and
she should practice safe sex, but I don't think she believes me. She believes she
will be rid of the HIV infection when the curse is removed. **How can I show
respect for her cultural beliefs but ensure she gets the treatment she
needs?**

This case may present one of the most difficult challenges to a
nurse's obligation to respect cultural differences, for this patient has
rejected one of the concepts that establish the basis for nursing practice, the Western ideas about the causes of infectious diseases. There
are two issues here: the patient's beliefs are influencing her to refuse
treatment for herself, and, more importantly, her beliefs stand in the
way of being willing to take steps to prevent harm to others by trans-
mitting the disease. The challenge is to determine which nursing interventions may succeed in getting her to understand the nature of the
disease, yet demonstrate respect for her cultural perspective.

Ideally, nurses are nonjudgmental, provide care without prejudice,
and value culturally diverse perspectives. Instead of rejecting the
patient's beliefs, the nurse should seek further information through a
cultural assessment, which would help to adequately identify the
patient's views about illness and treatment. A more comprehensive
view of the patient's cultural beliefs could help the nurse to find culturally appropriate explanations and suggestions that may persuade
the patient to accept the treatment she needs.

Second, patients who believe that illness results from the curses of
enemies or witch doctors may view Western medicine and treatments
as irrelevant and ineffective. If patients reject Western concepts about
the causes of their illness, they will understandably reject the appropriate treatment and may endanger their health substantially when

they forego medications designed to address physical causes while relying on cultural practices. Nurses have the obligation to educate patients about these risks and to attempt to persuade them that Western treatments are relevant and effective for treating these illnesses.

The most significant issue if patients reject Western concepts about the causes and treatment of infectious diseases arises when patients engage in behavior that endangers others, such as exposing them to HIV. This possibility imposes a stringent obligation on the nurse to redouble her efforts to educate this patient about the route of transmission of this disease, the effectiveness of Western treatment, and the necessity of protecting her sex partners. Ultimately, if others are at risk because a patient refuses treatment and does not modify the behavior that poses harm to others, the appropriate health agencies must be contacted.

Case 54

I have an elderly Puerto Rican patient who is refusing to take her blood pressure medications. She's already been hospitalized twice because her blood pressure was out of control. She told me she won' t take the prescribed medication because it's a "cold" medicine. She wants a "hot" medicine. **What should I do when a patient rejects necessary medical treatment because of cultural beliefs about medicines?**

This patient is rejecting standard medical treatment because she believes she needs a treatment that accords with her cultural traditions. Culturally competent nurses will know that certain cultures subscribe to a hot-cold theory of diseases, which holds that health requires a balance of hot and cold elements. Ideally, nurses would perform an initial assessment to ascertain a patient's cultural beliefs about the causes of illness and the treatments that are compatible with patients' cultural ideas. Based on this assessment, the nurse could then use the distinctions the patient draws and ask the physician about substitute medications that will fulfill the requirements of the patient's hot-cold theory of disease. Advocating treatments that are compatible with patients' cultural ideas is culturally competent care.

When the patient's cultural ideas are not compatible with Western medicine, nurses could encourage patients to discuss the situation with their families. Sometimes a member of the family can explain the proposed treatments and persuade patients to adopt a treatment or find a reasonable compromise that successfully protects the patient's health. In many communities, cultural groups exist that could also be contacted for suggestions.

Provided others are not at risk, when a patient has adequate information and competently makes a choice to reject treatment—any treatment—that choice must be respected. In that event, nurses should establish that a patient understands the nature of an illness and the efficacy of the recommended treatment, together with the risks of rejecting treatment. Because this patient has been hospitalized twice, the consequences of refusing blood pressure medication should be clear to her. Given that she is risking her life by rejecting the prescribed medication, it is imperative to exert all efforts to explain and educate her, though in the final analysis she may still refuse to take it.

Case 55

Russian families have recently moved into our community; they have a sponsor who sets them up in a house, maybe three families in an apartment. I have an elderly Russian patient with Type 2 diabetes which was diagnosed through a screening program the Department of Health runs. Her diabetes is worsening because it is impossible to get her to eat the proper diet. She eats one main meal a day from a large pot of food that's been cooking all day. All the families in her apartment share the same food. This is how she's been eating her whole life and she refuses to change. **What should I do when a diabetic refuses to give up her traditional foods?**

Patients who need special diets, such as diabetics, often resist recommendations to give up favorite foods and continue to eat whatever they please. This problem is exacerbated when they are advised to avoid foods that are an important part of their cultural traditions. Accepting a modified diet may seem like a minor change to make in order to have continued good health, but when that involves giving up cultural traditions, a patient may view this as an insurmountable challenge. Respect for cultural differences requires special attention to the need to develop diets that are adapted to the typical cultural preferences of patients. A patient's plan of care should include any dietary restrictions or cultural preferences.

The nurse could negotiate with this patient to develop a better diet that includes modified versions of traditional foods or perhaps refer the patient to a nutritionist. Though nurses can educate, counsel, persuade, and provide appropriate referrals, there is little else that they can do. Ultimately, the patient has the right to make the decision to continue with her traditional diet, even against her best interest.

Case 56

Cambodians and the Hmong practice coining. They use a coin to rub heated oil into the skin over the area that hurts, and then they place a glass over it. This leaves discolorations, but it reportedly is not painful. I have a case where a child needs to be hospitalized, but her family practices coining and rejects the doctor's advice. **Does this count as child abuse, or are these cultural beliefs protected by the law?**

Nurses are legally required in all states to report suspected cases of child abuse and neglect. There are, however, legal protections afforded to parents whose cultural practices can be construed as religious in nature. Many states have statutes exempting religiously motivated parents from being found guilty of child abuse and neglect for failing to secure traditional medical treatment for their children. Nevertheless, this case should be reported because the child's condition warrants hospitalization. It is the role of state agencies or courts, not nurses or physicians, to decide how to apply the legal exceptions.

ACCOMMODATING CULTURAL DIFFERENCES

Case 57

A patient of mine is a Navajo, an elderly man brought up in the traditions of the Navajo community who is being treated for cancer. Due to the chemotherapy he is receiving, his immune system is severely compromised. He is planning on having a traditional healing ceremony anyway. I'm concerned about his risk of infection if he is exposed to that many people. **Should I try to stop this?**

Perhaps more common than patients who reject Western practices completely are those who accept Western treatments but, at the same time, maintain their own cultural practices. The significance of a traditional healing ceremony should not be underestimated, since a patient's identity and values are defined, to some extent, by participation in cultural practices. As long as these practices do not pose a certain, imminent and serious harm, these traditions should be respected and accommodated to the extent that is compatible with Western nursing and medical practice. In fact, the Joint Commission on Accreditation of Healthcare Organizations requires healthcare facilities to include cultural needs, such as dietary restrictions, cultural beliefs and practices, when developing a plan of care for a patient.

A dilemma arises when cultural practices pose a risk to a patient's health. Nurses then face two moral requirements: the mandate to provide culturally competent care and the responsibility to protect a patient's health. These obligations can both be met if the traditional practices can be rendered compatible with the clinical advice of Western practitioners. The Navajo patient is in fact fully cooperating with standard Western treatment protocols, but he also wishes to participate in the healing ceremony important in his tradition. He may be convinced to postpone the ceremony until his immune system has recovered. If that is not feasible, he could perhaps be persuaded to wear a surgical mask to protect him from infection, or to restrict the number of people attending the healing ceremony to limit his exposure to germs. Unless he is willing to do this, the nurse should recommend against his participation at this time, for her obligation to patient safety and health takes precedence over the requirement to provide culturally competent care.

Case 58

> In my practice I've encountered several issues because some patients from other cultures don't accept our ideas about patient rights. One of my patients is an elderly Chinese man who needs to make a decision about his treatment. I can't get him to tell me what he wants to do. I've learned that I have to talk to his eldest son who is making all the decisions. **How can I be certain that a patient consents to treatment when the patient says nothing?**

Based on her professional obligation to protect patient rights, the nurse should advocate for this man's right to consent to treatment. This accords with an emphasis on individual decision-making and the rights of patients that permeates Western ideals of ethical nursing practice. However, patients from cultures where their personal lives are organized around strong social communities and complex family networks may not place the same value on those ideals. Accommodating some cultural practices may thus appear to require violating important ethical standards of individual rights.

The appropriateness of an ethical focus on the rights of separate individuals is already challenged by the realities of home health care. In this setting, the patient is usually best understood as an individual established within significant relationships, as an individual within a family, for example. Instead of acting as separate individuals, home health care patients may respond to illness as members of a more or less unified group and assign decision-making authority to someone else, abandon claims to confidentiality of information, and, in other ways, cede the individual rights afforded by Western traditions.

In general, patients have beliefs about family relationships and the roles and responsibilities of individuals within families that are influenced by their cultural values and standards. Patients from some cultural backgrounds expect their families to be present throughout convalescence or even when nurses and physicians examine them and discuss their care. In other cultures, the patient's "family" could include a whole clan or religious community, and this whole "family" could expect to help nurture someone back to health or to be present when the patient makes an exit from this world. Western ideals that emphasize individual patient rights to privacy and confidentiality of personal medical information appear to conflict with these cultural expectations. This conflict can be addressed by determining if a patient willingly accepts these practices and agrees to relinquish individual claims to privacy and confidentiality. If that is the case, these cultural practices accord with Western ideals that respect patient rights, by acknowledging that patients can waive these rights if they wish.

The ethical and legal requirements for informed consent, an important individual right, assume that competent adult patients will make decisions for themselves. Within communal societies, though, individuals may accept the decisions and wishes of the family or the group as their own. Also, in some cultures, gender roles and expectations require husbands to make decisions for their wives. Other cultures expect the young adult members of a family to defer to the decisions of the oldest male in the family or to accept the decisions of a nonrelated elder in the community. These cultural practices can be reconciled with the requirement that patients be allowed to make their own decisions if patients willingly acquiesce in assigning decision-making authority to others. For, although patients have the right to decide for themselves, they also have the right to waive their rights or to assign the right to make medical decisions to someone else, if they want to do so. Determining whether someone is freely ceding this right can be difficult, nonetheless, for there are no formal guidelines that can be used. Consequently, when someone other than the patient has assumed the responsibility to make decisions, it is important to assess whether the patient appears to agree with this and to offer the patient an opportunity to assent or dissent from any decisions that are made.

Finally, in the home health care context, paying attention to the patient's relationships to family and others in his community, and the consequences nursing actions have for those relationships, is imperative. Insisting on an individual's informed consent when it conflicts with cultural expectations, for example, could have harmful consequences for relationships that are valuable to a patient.

Knowledge of cultural beliefs about decision making and the significance of individual privacy and confidentiality of information are essential to the provision of culturally competent care. Accordingly, in their initial assessment of a patient's needs, nurses should determine whether a patient wants to designate someone to make his decisions for him, provide a patient the opportunity to waive rights, such as informed consent or privacy, and document these conversations. Certainly, in Case 58, the elderly Chinese patient can transfer his right to make medical decisions. The nurse should provide a chance for the patient to express his approval or disagreement with those decisions to ascertain that he has voluntarily assigned decision-making rights to his son. The patient's tacit acceptance may then be interpreted as his agreement with the choices made.

Case 59

I have found that some Portuguese families often do not want patients to know how sick they are. When family members are asked to translate medical information, they do not seem to interpret everything you're telling them. This is really a problem when a patient is terminally ill and it is important to know what their wishes are about end-of-life treatment. **What should I do when a patient's cultural values conflict with the duty to provide full disclosure of medical information?**

The moral and legal doctrine of informed consent requires health professionals to provide adequate and truthful information to individuals in order to facilitate an informed decision. The Patient Self-Determination Act also recognizes a patient's right to comprehensive information. Cultural values, however, may conflict with this requirement to address illness directly and openly with a patient. Some cultures expressly forbid disclosing information about a terminal illness or impending death. They believe that truthful information about the seriousness of an illness will cause a patient to lose hope, and thus they discourage sharing bad news with patients. Instead, families expect to hear the news first, and then decide what to tell the patient. Other cultures believe that words have the power to cause events. Telling a patient about the possible serious side-effects of a treatment, for example, is believed to have the power to cause those risks to become reality. For that reason, those cultures forbid disclosing full information about harmful consequences, including the possibility of impending death.

The standards utilized in determining whether the legal requirement of informed consent has been met have an undeniably Western bias. The law has traditionally ignored the fact that some individuals either do not want certain information or defer decision making to another family member, the community, or the authority of the physician. Recently, there has been a shift toward legally recognizing the values held by individual patients and the way these values are likely to influence medical decision making. Courts have held that, although the standard used must be objective, it must consider the needs of a reasonable person with all the characteristics of the plaintiff, including idiosyncrasies and religious beliefs. In addition, commissions that accredit healthcare organizations, such as the Joint Commission for Accreditation of Healthcare Organizations, now require all facilities to provide care that respects individuals' cultural values.

Therefore, patients from a cultural background in which the direct discussion of disease and death is anathema should not be forced to confront these realities if they do not wish to do so. In circumstances where information must be translated by families, it is appropriate to allow patients and families to follow their own cultural practices in such matters. When cultural values militate against full disclosure, nurses could encourage families to provide more information than is typical so that a patient's wishes for end-of-life treatment could be ascertained. But they should not reject the culturally accepted practices, unless they have good reason to believe that these practices endanger the patient's well-being or the patient objects and indicates that he wishes to assert his right to informed consent.

Case 60

One of my patients is near death. Because of her religious views, she believes she must maintain a state of awareness as death approaches and does not want to be heavily sedated or unconscious. She has bone cancer and is clearly in a lot of pain, but she refuses any pain medication except aspirin. Her son can hardly bear to visit her, and I have to admit I find it very difficult to be with her. **What should I do when a patient's religious beliefs conflict with my goal to relieve her suffering?**

The belief that pain is something to be avoided is so much a part of how most people respond to suffering that this patient may appear to be irrational. Though many dying patients will choose to forgo the kind of total pain relief that leaves them virtually comatose and unable to interact with their family and friends, they will still accept significant pain medication. It is thus unusual to care for patients who seem to welcome pain. Some patients believe that pain is ennobling and think that, if they can endure the pain, they will be better people. Others may think of pain as a kind of spiritual purification like the self-denial of observing fast days or engaging in certain religious practices that involve physical flagellation or self-inflicted pain. Still others may have guilt feelings about some action in the past and think of their pain as God's punishment for sin, something that is deserved.

Culturally competent care requires respect for patients' religious beliefs and skill in accommodating those beliefs in developing a plan of care. Therefore, this patient's right to refuse pain medication in accordance with her religious views should be respected. Nonetheless, given that this refusal appears to be against the patient's best interest, the nurse should initiate a discussion of the patient's reasons for this decision. The nurse could also suggest a visit from her religious leader to clarify what her religion requires. If the patient seems to have coherent, well-thought-out reasons consistent with her own values, her continued refusal of pain medications should be treated as any other instance of competent patients refusing treatment. To attempt to relieve her suffering, the nurse can suggest other nursing interventions which do not involve additional medications.

At the same time, the patient presumably would care about the effects on her son and the others around her when they are forced to watch her suffer so intensely. Although it is appropriate to mention the effect her behavior has on others, especially her son, this should not be presented as the deciding factor which should determine her choices. No one should use "emotional blackmail" to get patients to accept treatment.

Case 61

I have a new patient, an elderly man. When I first saw him, he was in bed, wearing only one slipper. I tried to remove it and he took offense. Actually, he got very upset, but he wouldn't tell me why. I later found out that he is an Orthodox Jew, and he is not supposed to be touched by a female who is not a member of his immediate family. **Should I have known that? Is it my obligation to know details about my patient's religious beliefs?**

Culturally competent care requires nurses to have knowledge of the taboos that are important to people of the cultures and religions that may be encountered in their practice. Taboos may include certain foods, such as pork products, which are an ingredient in some medications, or oyster shells, sometimes used in calcium supplements. Other taboos forbid care of females by male healthcare professionals, or restrict touching by others, as an example.

Culturally competent care begins with an initial assessment of a patient's cultural needs, including information about taboo foods, medicines, treatments, and practices, and these needs should be documented and accommodated in developing a plan of care. A cultural assessment should have revealed the patient's religious affiliation. Those with the responsibility to assign nurses to cases must know the basic requirements and restrictions of the major religious and ethnic groups within the agency's area. Given his religious affiliation, a female nurse should not have been assigned to care for this patient; hence, the agency is at fault for putting this nurse in this position, possibly because the agency supervisor did not know the patient's religious affiliation or did not understand the religious taboos that would affect nursing care. If the agency had no male nurse it could assign, this should have been discussed before the agency agreed to provide home health care for this patient. It could be necessary to refer a patient to another agency to ensure that the patient receives care that does not violate any religious prohibitions.

Nurses themselves also have a responsibility to know common religious taboos that are relevant to their nursing practice and to incorporate this cultural information into their care. Even where there is no preliminary cultural information that indicates the nurse must accommodate specific values or taboos, nurses should be sensitive to the possibility that cultural differences exist that may impact the planned nursing care. When a patient reacts unexpectedly to a gesture or comment, nurses should explore the possibility that a cultural or religious taboo has been violated and respond accordingly.

Case 62

Different cultures may have very different ideas about birthing practices and child-rearing. I see this in my practice because I do obstetrical work; I have a specialization in lactation. I recently told a Hmong patient that her baby was beautiful. When she responded with shock and asked me to leave, I found out that some Hmong families don't want us calling the baby "beautiful" because an evil spirit might hear and steal the baby's soul. **How can I avoid violating a patient's taboos?**

The taboo on calling a baby "beautiful" would be unexpected to anyone unfamiliar with Hmong traditions. This underscores the importance of developing adequate knowledge of the values, beliefs and practices of the cultural groups encountered in a nurse's practice. Initial cultural assessments should carefully explore the possibility that unexpected taboos or restrictions exist, to avoid violations of important cultural ideas. Nurses assigned to a patient's care should be briefed if there are religious or cultural taboos that must be avoided. Where there is no information about cultural restrictions, or there is doubt about the patient's preferences, nurses can usually avoid violating unknown taboos if they explain what they are about to do and ask permission.

It is also important to recognize that, even though specific cultural groups maintain characteristic values, beliefs, and practices, individuals may not accept all of the ideas attributed to their cultural group. Assuming that a person who is a member of a certain ethnic, religious, or national group will share all of the traditions of that group is an unwarranted generalization. Factors such as patients' ages and the length of time in this country, whether they live within a cultural community or are acculturated, and the level of education they have attained can influence the values and practices they maintain. As a matter of fact, studies show that socioeconomic status is more important in predicting an individual's values than racial or ethnic differences. Middle-class families tend to think and behave more like other middle-class families than like others of their own cultural group.

THE LIMITS OF TOLERANCE

Case 63

The nurses are all arguing because no one wants to go there. The family is from Southeast Asia. For religious reasons, they believe you shouldn't kill anything. Roaches; won't kill them. You set up a sterile field and a roach walks across it. I told the patient I need to maintain a sterile field to give my treatment. **Aren't there some things that I should not have to tolerate?**

Though nurses should strive to be nonjudgmental about patients' values and respect cultural differences, there are cultural practices which clearly should not be tolerated. These include practices which pose a risk of serious and imminent harm to the patient or others, which must be reported to the nurse's supervisor and the appropriate agencies. When a situation poses a risk to the safety of the nurse herself, she is justified in asking to be removed from the case and suggesting that the agency terminate its contract with a patient.

Other situations may involve a conflict between the patient's cultural beliefs and the nurse's principles. Since nurses and other health care professionals typically come from social, economic, and often cultural backgrounds that are very different from many of their patients, they may find that patients' lifestyle choices and personal behavior conflict with their own values. Family relationships which privilege male relatives may offend a nurse's sense of the rights of women, for example, while the practices of other cultures that do not place the same premium on personal cleanliness could be offensive. These cultural differences must be tolerated and respected, and nurses must avoid judgmental attitudes that stigmatize patients from those cultures.

A different kind of conflict of values may occur if, for example, a nurse who is a vegetarian and an animal rights activist encounters a family whose culture recommends healing ceremonies involving ritualistic animal sacrifice. These cultural practices will be intolerable because they violate the nurse's personal values. When these conflicts occur, nurses have the right to request to be reassigned, depending on the requirements of agency policy, but they still have a duty to provide care until someone else can take over the case.

In Case 63, the impossibility of establishing a sterile field makes any treatment risky for the patient. The patient, of course, has the right to reject the need for a sterile field, as long as he understands the risks he is taking. This is not to imply that the nurse has no rights of her own. Surely she has a professional and moral right to insist on the minimal conditions for meeting nursing standards for providing care. If these conditions cannot be met, she may have to recommend that the agency withdraw from the case.

Case 64

> I've just discovered that one of my female patients was circumcised as a girl before she immigrated to this country. She looks back on it as a valuable rite of passage and an important way to stay connected to her culture. She has asked me if I can recommend a doctor who will circumcise her daughter in a safe, sterile way. **I'm dead set against this, but should I cooperate with her as a way of respecting her beliefs and values?**

This kind of situation raises the complicated question of ethical relativism. It is clear that what is considered permissible or even required in one culture may be considered wrong in another. Ethical relativism claims that these cultural views about right and wrong establish the moral code in a society. Actions considered right are actually right in that society, and actually wrong in societies that consider them wrong. Morality, according to this view, is different from place to place, time to time, and culture to culture. All cultural practices should, therefore, be tolerated, because these practices are right according to the standards of their own culture.

Contrary to the relativists' view, many believe some actions are genuinely wrong for all human beings, regardless of their cultural perspectives. Murder and torture are two examples of actions that are judged wrong for all cultures. Therefore, according to this view, there are some actions that should not be tolerated.

In the case of female circumcision, the United States legal system has determined that it is a practice that should not be tolerated. It is now illegal for anyone, doctors and nurses included, to participate in this practice. The nurse therefore should not cooperate in any way in perpetuating the practice in this country. She should be understanding of the cultural context in which her patient was raised, but at the same time do her best to dissuade her from her plan to have her daughter subjected to this procedure.

On the whole, it is easier to make the case that certain practices should not be tolerated if the subject is a child or an incompetent person. When the practice is freely engaged in by competent adults and is not illegal, their right to decide for themselves is paramount, even if it involves what others see as doing harm to themselves. However, they do not have the right to insist on the participation of nurses or others in these cultural practices.

ANALYSIS OF CASE 51

Case 51 involves a Haitian woman who believes she is suffering because she was cursed. Consequently, she has refused to take the prescribed medications and instead insists on a folk remedy she believes will cure her. The ethical issue is how the nurse should respond to this cultural practice.

First and foremost, the nurse's response to this situation must demonstrate sensitivity to the woman's cultural beliefs and respect for her cultural values. She should avoid dismissing or denigrating the patient's view about the actual cause of her physical condition, even though it contradicts Western understandings of the origin of the complications she suffered after giving birth.

As a competent adult, the patient has the right to make decisions based upon her own personal values and concerns, including her cultural beliefs. She therefore has the right to make the decision to reject Western medical practices in favor of cultural remedies, as long as she has been fully informed about the consequences of that decision and the decision is voluntary. The nurse's responsibility is to establish that the patient is well informed about the nature of her illness and the prescribed treatment, in order to validate her right to refuse the treatment.

Though the nurse is concerned about the patient's welfare, it would show a lack of respect for the patient's personal values simply to reject her beliefs about the effectiveness of the folk remedy and attempt to have her accept different values. Without disputing the patient's beliefs, the nurse may be able to persuade her to take the prescribed medication in addition to her folk remedy. To accomplish this, the nurse might be able to enlist the help of someone from the patient's cultural group or her family to discuss the need for the prescribed medications.

However, the nurse must also consider the consequences that may follow from the patient's insistence on the folk remedy. It is imperative to determine what the remedy contains to decide if it is harmful or would be harmful if taken together with the prescribed substance. If the remedy is harmful, or if it interferes with a necessary and effective treatment, the nurse should not support the use of the folk remedy and should ensure that the patient fully understands the harmful conse-quences of maintaining the cultural practice. Assuming that the Haitian patient's folk remedy is harmless, the nurse could support the patient's decision to take the remedy, while encouraging her to take advantage of the benefits of the prescribed medications.

Culturally competent nursing care begins with an assessment of the individual patient's cultural views about health and illness. Nurses must display respect for those cultural views, incorporate them into the patient's plan of care, and develop skills in accommodating cul-tural values when providing nursing care. Nurses must also be able to determine when cultural practices should not be tolerated.

ETHICAL CRITERIA

- Respect cultural differences.
- Recognize the limits of tolerance for cultural practices that are harmful or illegal.

PRACTICAL STRATEGIES

When patients are from diverse cultural backgrounds:

- Acquire knowledge about the preferences of religious and ethnic groups.

• Perform an assessment of cultural beliefs and values.

When patients reject Western practices:

• Determine whether the alternative treatment is harmful to the patient.
• Notify the physician if the alternative treatment or refusal of treatment is deemed harmful.
• Educate the patient about the nature of the illness and the goals of Western treatment.
• Suggest to the physician other Western treatments that would accommodate the patient's cultural and religious beliefs.

When a family's cultural beliefs impact the health of a child:

• Assess whether the child's health is jeopardized.
• Discuss concerns with the family.
• Report suspected instances of child abuse and neglect.

When competent, adult patients engage in cultural practices or religious healing rituals:

• Determine whether the practice will pose a threat of serious harm to the patient.
• Discuss concerns with the patient, if harm will result.
• Attempt to negotiate a compromise that will diminish the risks for the patient, while accommodating the religious or cultural practice.

When cultural practices limit individual patients' rights:

• Determine whether the patient has waived the right.
• Consider whether insisting on protecting individual rights will do more harm than good.

When religious or cultural beliefs may result in taboos:

• Explain the nursing role to the patient.
• Ask about specific restrictions based on religious and cultural practices or beliefs.

When cultural practices hinder the performance of nursing duties:

- Assess whether the patient is at risk.
- Determine whether the environment places the nursing staff at risk.
- Report cases where the patient or nurse is placed at risk.
- Discuss moral objections with your supervisor.
- Approach the agency's ethics committee for advice.

Chapter 7

FACING THE END OF LIFE

Patients who are terminally ill must often make difficult decisions about their treatment, decisions that their families may fail to understand or accept. As a result, nurses confront vexing ethical questions about their responsibilities, both to dying patients and to their families.

Case 65

My patient with end-stage cancer has finally decided he's through with all the treatments he's getting. He told his sons he doesn't want to continue. They don't understand why. They're pretty upset about this because they feel he is just giving up, and they're putting a lot of pressure on him to change his mind. Despite this, the patient has continued to insist that he wants no more treatment, and now he is saying that he doesn't want to be resuscitated if something happens to him. **Should I intervene if his sons try to overturn these decisions when he is no longer able to decide for himself?**

General Issues

- **What treatments do dying patients have a right to refuse?**
- **How should end-of-life decisions be made for incompetent patients?**
- **What is the nurse's responsibility to families when patients are dying?**
- **Do nurses have a responsibility to help patients achieve the kind of death they want?**

INTRODUCTION

When they are dying, patients may reject hospitalization and choose to remain at home, where they hope for a peaceful death, surrounded by family and friends. They may also expect to have more control over their final days in a home setting that seems to allow them to assert the authority to make their own decisions to the fullest extent. In reality, however, dying patients may actually have less control in this context. When a patient has decided to forgo heroic measures, for example, a hospital staff will respect that decision. But at home, families may panic when they face the prospect of death occurring and rush the dying person to the emergency room for treatment. On the other hand, if a patient decides at the end to reverse a previous decision to forgo heroics and instead seek aggressive treatment or resuscitation, this will be more difficult or even impossible to accomplish at home. More important, families are not always in full agreement with patients' decisions about life-sustaining treatment. Though they seem to accept a patient's decision, they may try to impose their own decisions once patients can no longer express their wishes.

Families who accept the responsibility of caring for a dying patient at home may find the actual experience of the dying process to be overwhelming. Despite the best intentions to provide loving care, they may find it so arduous and even disagreeable to give the care required for someone who is dying that they sometimes fail to follow the plan of care and may even neglect a patient. Family caregivers can thus create problems that ordinarily would not arise in a hospital or nursing home setting, where professional staff is always on call to ensure that the requisite care is provided for patients at the end of life.

Thus, the iconic image of dying at home, with control over one's final days, surrounded by family and friends who provide loving care and attention until a peaceful death occurs, is often quite different from the reality. The reality is that home health care nurses are caring for patients and families who are commonly depressed, anxious, physically exhausted, emotionally overwhelmed by the difficulties of facing the end of life, and sometimes in fundamental disagreement about the decisions that must be made.

THE RIGHTS OF DYING PATIENTS TO REFUSE TREATMENT

Case 66

I remember a man with metastatic thyroid cancer who was on an experimental chemotherapy protocol. The doctors didn't have any standard treatment to offer him. They were just trying to give him some hope by enrolling him in the protocol. He finally said "enough" and refused to go for any more treatments. **What is my responsibility to a patient who refuses the only available treatment?**

Though this dying patient has refused the only treatment his doctors can offer, that is his moral and legal right. Competent patients always have the right to decide whether to accept or reject any treatment for their illnesses, even when refusal means certain death. Moreover, the chemotherapy treatments appear to be futile in this case, and, in situations where further treatment is futile, that is, will not reverse the progress of a disease, prolong life, or offer any medical benefit, there is no moral obligation either to accept treatment or to administer treatment. The patient is clearly within his rights to reject this treatment.

One responsibility the nurse has is to support and protect the patient's right to make such decisions. When patients face vital decisions, nurses can provide important clarifications in response to questions about their health, help patients identify their options, and assist patients in articulating their own values. Nurses are often in a unique position to support patients and to act as advocates in these circumstances.

Most significantly, though the patient has refused experimental chemotherapy treatments, he has not rejected nursing care, which often plays a valuable role in achieving a good death. Nurses should aggressively advocate for all the supportive and palliative care they believe dying patients need. This is particularly important because some physicians may be inclined to abandon a patient who has rejected treatment aimed at curing his disease.

Hospice care may be appropriate for this patient. Patients are eligible to enter a program of hospice care when their illness is terminal and they are expected to live no longer than six months. Although its use tripled between 1991 and 2000, hospice care is still underutilized in this country. A surprising number of patients are admitted to hospice care only in the last three days of life. Most often the reason is that physicians are reluctant to make referrals, fearing that it will lead to a loss of hope. Sometimes patients or families are reluctant because they view the move to hospice as giving up, at a time when they want to do all they can to prolong life.

Actually, hospice care offers many benefits to terminally ill patients because it takes a holistic approach. In addition to nursing care services, hospice care offers expert palliative care and a whole spectrum of practical, emotional, and spiritual support for both the patient and the family. When patients are admitted to hospice care, they may decide to give up any therapy aimed at a cure, though that is no longer a condition of receiving hospice care. Even if they make that decision, the palliative care they receive can include radiation, blood transfusions, and even chemotherapy if the therapy will shrink a tumor which is causing pain.

Patients may receive hospice care at home, in a freestanding hospice facility, in a hospital, or in a nursing home. When home care and hospice are combined, the patient receives the benefit of continuity of care by the same nurse. Dying patients who prefer admission to a facility to remaining at home, perhaps because there are small children in the home, can choose a nursing home or freestanding hospice facility for hospice care. Even if the patient's condition requires hospitalization, the patient can still be cared for according to hospice philosophy in that setting.

Ideally, the patient's physician will suggest the move to hospice when he or she has made the judgment that a patient has six months or less to live. If a nurse concludes that the time may be right for hospice care, based on her professional assessment of a patient's situation and her conversations with the patient, she can convey this assessment to the patient's physician, who has the responsibility to make the judgment that a patient qualifies for this care. If the physician seems resistant to this suggestion, a nurse can also encourage a patient to discuss the plan of care with the physician, without directly mentioning hospice care.

Case 67

Some doctors do not address end-of-life decisions with their patients. I have a young woman who has refused all treatment. Her doctor is livid. He screamed at her: "You can live! This is nonsense!" He told me to try to get her to change her mind. But she is clear that she doesn't want anything else done. **Do I have an obligation to try to change her mind?**

When patients decide to refuse life-saving treatments, nurses should first attempt to confirm that the decision is a patient's own voluntary decision rather than a choice that has been imposed by the patient's family or others. If it is clear that this patient's decision is voluntary and informed, the question is whether it is then ethically acceptable to try to change her mind. Certainly it is always appropriate to initiate discussion, identify relevant facts, and appeal to values patients hold, in an effort to persuade them to undergo treatment. But once the patient's decision has been confirmed as voluntary, this is as far as any-one should go to try to affect the decision. This would satisfy a nurse's duty to follow a doctor's orders, even though the doctor may have wanted her to be more aggressive. Although the physician has asked the nurse to try to change the patient's mind, it would not be ethically acceptable to manipulate the patient or to attempt to dictate a deci-sion, even if it would seem to be in the best interest of the patient.

Finally, although nurses normally have an obligation to carry out a physician's order unless it appears to be in error, they also should chal-lenge an order when it seems patently unethical. Protecting the patient's right to decide about continuing treatment, even life-saving treatment, is the nurse's responsibility. This can require nurses to sup-port patients who have made decisions nurses themselves question. Some patients, nurses may believe, give up on treatment too soon, while others have unrealistic expectations and only prolong their suf-fering by deciding to endure further treatment. Nonetheless, it is still the patient's decision to make, even if doctors denounce the decision as nonsense.

DECIDING FOR INCOMPETENT PATIENTS

Case 68

One of my patients was a Comfort One patient who lived with her sister. She was being treated for complications from congestive heart failure. She under-stood that she could one day "crash" and she made it clear she didn't want to be resuscitated when that happened. We talked it over, and I thought her sister understood her decision. But when she developed breathing problems last week, her sister called me in a panic. I went over right away. She was unconscious when I got there and the Comfort One bracelet was missing. Her sister had called an ambulance. **Should I have tried to stop the paramedics from resuscitating her?**

While individuals are still competent, they can exercise the right to self-determination by expressing their wishes for end-of-life treatment, as this woman has done. A Living Will can state in general terms a person's wish to avoid the use of extraordinary means, such as a ventilator, to sustain life when an illness is terminal. Individuals who sign a Durable Power of Attorney for Health Care name someone else to make decisions for them in any situation in which they are unable to make their own decisions. For example, if an individual is unconscious and thus incompetent, the agent named in the document would have the authority to make medical decisions. This document can include specific instructions about which measures are to be accepted or omitted. Both of these documents, known as advance directives, carry legal weight and should determine a patient's end-of-life care when the patient has become incompetent. Without this documentation, the assumption is generally made that all life-sustaining measures should be taken.

Advance directives are particularly useful documents when patients are hospitalized and wish to refuse life-sustaining treatments. Home health care patients can usually forgo unwanted end-of-life treatment by simply avoiding the hospital, since the use of heroic measures to sustain life typically requires hospitalization.

The situation is complicated if someone decides to contact emergency medical personnel when a patient is dying at home. Until recently, if a family called for emergency assistance, the emergency medical technician (EMT) was required to resuscitate the patient even against the patient's or surrogate's wishes. In fact, even if a copy of a valid Living Will or Do Not Resuscitate (DNR) order were visible, the EMT had no legal authority to carry out the order to avoid resuscitation.

That has changed with recent legislation which permits emergency medical technicians to respect Allow Natural Death and DNR orders in the home health care setting. Comfort One bracelets, standard hospital bracelets with Allow Natural Death or DNR printed on them, authorize emergency medical personnel to carry out these orders. A request from a family member or friend does not override a valid DNR order signified by the fact that the patient is wearing a Comfort One bracelet or necklace.

The issuance of Comfort One bracelets emerged as a result of a legal progression that began with the 1990 United States Supreme Court decision in *Cruzan v Director, Missouri Department of Health*, which recognized a constitutionally-protected liberty right to refuse life-sustaining treatment. During the same year, Congress enacted the Patient Self-Determination Act (PSDA), affirming patients' rights to refuse medical treatment, even if death would result from the refusal. The PSDA applies to all health care facilities receiving Medicaid or Medicare funds and mandates (1) documentation in the patient's medical records of whether or not a medical directive has been executed; (2) education for the community and staff on issues concerning advance directives; (3) maintaining written policies and procedures to accept or refuse life-sustaining treatment and carry out advance directives; and (4) providing patients with written information about these policies.

Following the PSDA legislation, all states moved to authorize physicians to issue "do not resuscitate" orders for consenting patients. DNR orders are activated only in the event that an individual is incompetent to express his or her wishes. These orders originally applied only to health care facilities, which included hospitals and nursing homes. Later laws were amended to include hospices and to offer "portability" between hospitals, nursing homes, and hospices. This makes it possible for the orders to remain in effect if a patient requires being moved from one type of facility to another. A licensed home health care agency now falls within the category of "health care facility." This legislation, in turn, applies to licensed practical nurses, registered nurses, and other health care personnel who provide services in the patient's home. Thus, DNR orders are now recognized as being in force when a nurse is providing care in the home, as well as in hospitals and other health care facilities.

Most state statutes allow patients to revoke advance directives whether or not they are competent. Hence, an incompetent person may revoke a DNR order, even if the decision is not consistent with the decision the patient would have made if competent. Because of patents' rights in this regard, special provisions have been included in state legislation specifying procedures for notifying staff of each health care facility involved when a DNR order has been voluntarily revoked by the patient. Previously, a patient's revocation had to be communicated to a physician or nurse at a hospital, hospice, or nursing home. Now, the patient can communicate these wishes, verbally or otherwise, to any health care personnel, who are then responsible for immediately informing the physician of the revocation.

Case 69 illustrates the complexities of caring for dying patients who do not wish to be resuscitated. Though families cannot legally override a decision that a patient made while competent, they may try to do so if they disagree with that decision or if they simply panic as a patient nears death. An intact Comfort One bracelet would have guaranteed that this patient would not be resuscitated by the EMTs, no matter what her sister wanted. However, once the bracelet has been removed or tampered with in any way, the EMTs are required to resuscitate, unless a physician provides a DNR order. The nurse's legal options here are limited to contacting the patient's doctor to ask him to give the DNR order. From a moral perspective, she should continue to advocate following the patient's wishes when those wishes are known, as they were in this case.

Case 69

I have a patient who isn't able to make any decisions herself. She's a seventy-six-year-old demented woman who is dying. No one knows what she would want us to do. Should I just ask someone in her family to decide? **How should these decisions be made for her?**

When patients are unable to make their own decisions because they are unconscious or otherwise incompetent, a proxy decision maker is necessary. In the absence of specific instructions, nurses, physicians, and hospitals must turn to family members to give consent. There is no standard procedure for determining who the decision maker should be, though usually a spouse, partner, adult child, or a parent, in the case of a young child, takes on that role. Problems can arise if the family disagrees about who should decide or disagrees about the decision itself. In these circumstances nurses should encourage family discussion until agreement or consensus is reached, if possible. A legal determination of the appropriate decision maker may be needed if a decision involves life and death consequences.

Proxy decision makers should use the standard of substituted judgment, which requires making the decision the patient would have made in cases where the patient expressed her own wishes about treatment while she was competent. Advance directives or statements a patient made in earlier conversations can be used to determine what the patient would have wanted. If there is uncertainty about a patient's wishes for treatment, a nurse should ask the family about any conversations they might have had with the patient about similar situations and document any relevant information concerning the patient's values and wishes. Generally, nurses should always document any discussions they have with patients in which they identify their wishes for end-of-life treatment. If there is no evidence of patient preferences, or if the patient was never competent, then the proxy uses the best interest of the patient standard. The best interest standard is applied by choosing as a reasonable person would be expected to choose under the circumstances. This may be determined by weighing the costs and benefits of the available options.

In addition to treatment decisions on behalf of a patient, a proxy decision maker is allowed to make the decision to stop treatment at the end of life. It should be noted here that there is no moral difference between decisions to withhold treatment and decisions to withdraw treatment already initiated. If it would have been ethically acceptable to decide against initiating treatment in the first place, then it is felt to be acceptable to withdraw treatment when that treatment proves to be ineffective, futile, or very burdensome to the patient. There is often, of course, a pronounced psychological difference between deciding not to start treatment and "pulling the plug." Yet, the intention and the effect are the same: the underlying disease or medical condition will progress until the patient succumbs. While difficult, these decisions should be made on the same basis as other proxy decisions, that is, on the basis of substituted judgment where that is possible, or, alternatively, using the best interest of the patient to determine the course of action.

Case 70

I've been caring for a man who had a stroke and a heart attack during surgery and is clearly not recovering. He has occasional periods of consciousness and does feel pain, but he is basically uncommunicative and has some paralysis as a result of his stroke. His wishes about treatment are unknown. The patient's daughter cannot accept what has happened and keeps saying that she wants the doctors to "do everything." **What should I say when families say "do everything," but I know further treatment is futile?**

Families who must make decisions for an incompetent patient whose wishes are unknown often invoke the phrase "Do everything." It is important to think about the motivation behind this. Although this is phrased as a decision, it functions more like a slogan or an emotional outburst. Only a careful discussion will reveal what families really mean. Does the family believe that recovery is possible, and is there any evidence that this is true? Or, if it is clear that this is a false belief, is it based on simple denial, a refusal to believe that the end is near? Is it based on guilt and the thought that the decision to "do everything" demonstrates love and devotion? Is it based on a confused idea that withdrawing treatment is tantamount to killing the patient?

Although the physician has the responsibility to inform the family about the patient's prognosis when the patient is incompetent, distraught families often do not "hear" this information and may have false beliefs about the possibility of recovery. Nurses may need to clarify information, answer questions, and initiate discussion to assess the family's understanding of the patient's prognosis when families want to "do everything" for patients like this man. Nurses can also help families to cope with emotions such as guilt by explaining that the decision to "do everything" is not required to demonstrate love and devotion. Families express love through the decisions they make for a dying patient when those decisions are based on the values that person held dear, or when they make choices that advance the best interest of the patient. In situations where continuing treatment is causing the patient more suffering than benefit, the family can demonstrate their love through acting to reduce the patient's suffering by withdrawing treatment.

If it is clear that further treatment is futile, that is, will not provide any medical benefit, this must be explained to the family. Nurses may also help to clarify the situation when there is no way to improve the patient's quality of life, even with treatment, and he will not in any meaningful sense return to being the person he once was. Families will find their end-of-life decisions eased by the understanding that, from an ethical point of view, there is no requirement that futile treatments be provided. More importantly, the nurse should assure the family that stopping treatment does not mean withdrawing nursing care or abandoning a patient.

Finally, the nurse should assure the family that withdrawing treatment is allowing the natural course of events to unfold; it is not tantamount to killing the patient. In these circumstances the patient is dying from the underlying physical problems. Withdrawing treatment is what some have called "passive euthanasia," which has become widely accepted as ethical practice. "Active euthanasia," i.e., acting to cause death, such as giving a lethal dose of medication with the intent to cause death, is legally wrong in this country, and is clearly prohibited by the ethical standards of professional nursing.

Case 71

I had a two-year-old patient with cancer. His parents knew he was dying, but they were willing to do everything that would prolong his life as long as he wasn't in pain. At the end, though, he was in a lot of pain. I still remember his mother saying to me: "Can't we just put an end to his suffering?" I gave the morphine dose that was prescribed, but I could lose my license if I gave an extra dose, and I knew the doctor would not prescribe more. **Is there anything else I could have ethically done to end his suffering?**

The unrelieved suffering of a dying child underscores the need for nurses and families to aggressively advocate for better pain management for patients. Numerous recent studies show that both adults and children are seriously undermedicated at the end of life, with children suffering even more than adults. There may be several reasons for the undermedication of children, including false information about the ability of infants and young children to feel pain, skepticism when an older child reports pain, and a fear that the use of pain medication may lead to addiction. None of these are sufficient reasons to allow a dying child to suffer.

Because he would not prescribe an increased dose of morphine, this physician was apparently acting on the basis of an accepted standard of practice that limits medication which could be seen as hastening death. This standard of practice should be challenged. Larger doses of pain medication could be justified by appealing to the principle of double effect. According to this moral principle, an action which has both good and bad effects could be justified if the intention is to accomplish good, and the bad effect is a foreseen but unintended result. In this case, administering high doses of pain medication would be intended to alleviate pain, though it is known that large doses of morphine will result in depressed respiration, which could contribute to an earlier death. If larger doses of morphine were prescribed, the nurse could ethically administer the drug, given that the American Nurses' Association (ANA) Code of Ethics advises that nurses should provide interventions intended to relieve pain even when this entails a risk of hastening death.

The nurse could also have recommended the family discuss hospice care with the physician. This is a good option when the main issue is pain control, since hospice care introduces expertise in palliative care. The primary focus and experience of hospice nurses and physicians is on the relief of pain and the control of symptoms at the end of life, which would clearly have benefited this child. In addition, given the resources of hospice programs, they would have been able to provide more comprehensive support for the family than it would be possible for the nurse to do on her own.

RESPONSIBILITIES TO FAMILIES WHEN PATIENTS ARE DYING

Case 72

I have a patient, a lung cancer patient, who doesn't want to be treated any longer. His wife and sons are in denial and they want treatment, so he's going along with them. This is really making things worse. He is getting sick from the chemotherapy and I know he wants to stop, but he doesn't want his family to know how much he's hurting. Even though he could have a much better quality of life without the chemotherapy, he won't let me talk to them about it. **Should I tell his family he is trying to hide what the treatment is doing to him, in order to spare them?**

This patient's treatment decisions demonstrate his overriding concern for his family. Patients' relationships, especially the intimate connections patients seek to maintain with their families and others who are valuable and integral parts of their lives, exert emotionally powerful influences on their end-of-life decisions. Patients may make certain choices or conceal information because of their concern about the effect on their families. They may fear that honest disclosures about their feelings and experiences will have an adverse impact on a relationship, and they may wish to protect significant others from as much sadness and emotional pain as possible. Consequently, when ethical questions arise about the end-of-life decisions patients have made, their relationships are an essential factor to consider.

The nurse's dilemma in Case 72 arises from a conflict between two ethical commitments: the nurse's obligation to respect a competent patient's own decisions supports withholding information from his family. However, the nurse's overall obligation to a patient's welfare supports telling them how much harm the treatments are doing. Does one of these commitments take precedence? The best approach to solving this dilemma is to attend to all of the dimensions of the patient's individual situation, including his relationships.

First, the nurse can meet the requirement to respect a patient's right to make his own decisions by discussing these ethical concerns directly with the patient and encouraging him to find a way to tell his family his true feelings. She could offer to facilitate this discussion with his family by talking with them first, in general terms, to prepare them for his dying. If he consents to disclosure of the true nature of his situation, the frank discussion could result in his family's support for a decision to end chemotherapy, which would result in a better quality of life for the patient.

Nevertheless, a nurse should not reveal the patient's feelings about treatment without the patient's approval. That is the only way to respect both his decision to spare his family and his right to determine who has access to medical information. This approach also allows a dying patient to satisfy the psychological need to maintain some control over his situation.

Should the overall obligation to promote the patient's well-being yield to these ethical commitments to respect patient self-determination and confidentiality? In fact, a comprehensive view of the patient's welfare would take into account his need to have some control, his wish to protect his family, and his desire to weight the consequences for his family above any concerns about his own well-being. His welfare, that is, is inseparable from these significant psychological and emotional needs; thus any appraisal of his welfare must recognize his primary concern for his family. In the final analysis, a complete assessment of this patient's particular situation reveals that there is no real conflict in this case between the obligations to respect the patient's right to self-determination and to promote patient welfare. Therefore, the nurse should not disclose the information about the effects of the chemotherapy or the patient's wish to stop treatment.

Case 73

A patient with cancer wants as much chemotherapy as the doctors will give her, even after her own doctor said there is nothing more he can do. She wants more, more, more. Her husband wants her to spend more time with their children, but she's too busy running to new doctors. He wants her to say "I've had enough" because he's had enough. He complains to me about it. I don't think she believes she is really that sick. **If a patient's denial is hurting her family, what would I be justified in doing?**

This patient's denial is not an uncommon response to a terminal illness, especially in the early stages. According to many psychologists, individuals then advance through other stages until reaching a peaceful state of acceptance of death. However, though a common response to death in Western culture, this should not become a prescription for how people ought to think and feel about dying. Because people have distinct personalities, values, religious and ethnic traditions, and diverse experiences with death and dying, they will approach dying in their own individual ways. Nurses should respect a patient's individual approach to dying, given that the right of self-determination presumably includes the right to determine how to cope with death, including the denial of impending death. Where there are serious concerns that a patient is clinically depressed, the nurse should recommend depression screening to the physician and, if appropriate, a referral for counseling services. Patients, of course, have the right to refuse these interventions and to continue coping with dying in their own individual ways.

This patient's denial and relentless pursuit of further treatment is exacting serious costs for her family. Certainly she has a right to make her own decisions in response to her terminal illness, but the significant consequences for her husband and children raise the question of the extent of the responsibilities a nurse has to a patient's family. Though a nurse's primary responsibility is to the patient, nursing care is also directed at meeting the comprehensive needs of patients' families, as the ANA Code of Ethics establishes. Because the patient may not be aware of the effects of her actions on her husband and children, the nurse should encourage a family discussion. She could also suggest the process of shared decision-making, which would provide the opportunity to address the interests of all of them. Another option is for the nurse to attempt to minimize the negative consequences of the patient's unending quest for more treatment. For example, she should encourage the patient to interact with her children in ways that do not interfere with her own efforts to obtain treatment. In these ways the nurse can be an advocate for the patent's family but also respect the patient's wish to approach her dying in her own way.

Case 74

Sometimes patients know what they want, but their families don't agree. I had a forty-five-year-old dialysis patient. She was alert, oriented, functional, but she had just had it when she decided not to continue with dialysis. Her family had real trouble dealing with this. Although I was upset, too, I was especially concerned about the effects on her family. **What exactly is my responsibility to a family when a patient decides to give up treatment?**

Though competent patients have the right to make the decision to stop dialysis treatments, others may find it hard to imagine that any life-sustaining treatment is not worth the effort. For some, rejecting treatment such as dialysis is tantamount to suicide. Consequently, when patients "just give up," the effect on their families is often devastating. Families may respond with accusations of "suicide," feelings of abandonment, and real anger at the patient. The resulting bitterness may prevent the sort of personal experiences that are important to dying patients and their families. It is clear that family relationships may be seriously and perhaps irreparably damaged when families disagree with the decision to stop treatment.

Nurses should help families to distinguish a decision to refuse a treatment that is necessary for sustained existence from the act of suicide. When life-sustaining treatment is refused, the underlying physiological condition, as opposed to the patient's own action, is the cause of death. In contrast, suicide is the intentional taking of one's own life, where the patient does something to cause his or her own death, which would not otherwise occur at that time. Death can be intentionally brought about through omissions as well as actions. In fact, it is estimated that the death of many elderly patients can be attributed to refusing to eat, "forgetting" to take medications, or "mistakenly" taking an overdose.

One responsibility the nurse has in Case 74 is to help the patient understand the effects her decision has on her family. She could offer to facilitate a family discussion of the burdens of dialysis treatment and the patient's reasons for deciding to stop treatment. This would also give family members the opportunity to express their concerns and frustrations with this decision. In addition, if the patient seems uncertain about what to do, a nurse could also encourage her to involve her family in shared decision-making. This process may lead to better understanding and help to minimize the negative consequences when a family disapproves of the patient's decision.

The nurse also has the important responsibility to support the family as they try to come to terms with this decision, providing them with information and answering questions about the patient's health, with the patient's consent. She could also recommend that a social worker become involved to provide in-depth counseling, as needed.

Finally, though nurses have the responsibility to attempt to meet the comprehensive needs of the patient's family when patients decide to reject life-sustaining treatment, they must continue to support the patient's right to make this decision, no matter how difficult that is for families to accept.

Case 75

I have a patient, a widow who is living with her daughter and her family. She has Alzheimer's. When I go into the home I see the uneasiness. Everyone is so stressed. I spend so much time trying to make peace. The patient has just been diagnosed with breast cancer. Her daughter and son don't want her to have any treatment for the cancer because they are sure they know what their mother would want. Her granddaughter is horrified, though. When I got there today she was screaming at them. She wants me to help her get treatment for her grandmother. **What should I do when families disagree about treatment?**

The key to resolving such family disagreements may lie in having the family review the justification for the decision to refuse treatment. The first step is to identify and evaluate the reasons for the decision. The most compelling reason for a particular decision regarding an incompetent patient, like this one, is direct evidence of the patient's own wishes, such as previous comments or information about the values that were important to the patient. When such information is available, the decision could be justified by appealing to the standard of substituted judgment.

If the patient has not addressed the question of forgoing treatment while competent, the decision could still be justified by considering the consequences of treatment versus nontreatment and making a decision based on the best interest of the patient. With any of the standard treatments, depending on how advanced the cancer is, the burdens are likely to be substantial, and, for a patient who cannot understand the purposes of treatment, the burdens are increased. Hence, the goal of avoiding additional suffering could justify nontreatment as a good option. On the other hand, if the care would be palliative in some way, for example, removing a large mass pressing on vital organs, then the benefits might outweigh the burdens. In that case, a decision to refuse the treatment may not be justified. A review of the reasons, burdens and benefits that can justify the decision to refuse treatment should help resolve the disagreement between family members, though even when families have reached agreement on what should be done, they will often find the decision to forgo treatment for a dying patient emotionally difficult.

The decision to reject treatment for someone else would fail to be justified when the reasons for making the decision are weak or outright unethical. Decisions based primarily on the grandmother's age, for example, could constitute age discrimination, which is both immoral and illegal. Similarly, when the refusal is based simply on the fact of dementia, that refusal may be difficult to justify. Likewise, if a treatment is very effective and not burdensome, such as taking antibiotics for an infection, a decision not to treat is controversial. Finally, if personal interests such as inheritance are motivating a family rather than the welfare of the patient, the decision to refuse treatment cannot be justified.

Nurses should encourage family discussions to foster consensus about the treatment decisions that must be made, if possible, and provide the resources and support necessary to family members, such as this granddaughter, who do not accept the family decision. Some nurses will be able to facilitate a family discussion themselves. Nurses could also suggest that the family involve a social worker, counselor, or clergy who can fulfill that role.

HELPING PATIENTS ACHIEVE THE KIND
OF DEATH THEY WANT

Case 76

> One of my AIDS patients is fifty years old. He lives alone. His family doesn't know he is gay. They think he has cancer and they want to know why he isn't getting chemotherapy. He is finding it harder to keep the truth from them now, because he is developing multiple opportunistic infections and his condition is worsening. He realizes he is dying and has recently decided that he wants no more secrets between them. He wants to tell them he is gay, and he wants me to help him talk to them and answer their questions. **How much should I do to help a dying patient take care of unfinished business?**

Dying patients often face emotional and psychological crises that may prevent a peaceful death, such as the emotional pain of unresolved family conflicts or the urgency of the desire to reconcile with significant others and family members who are estranged. Given the ideal expressed by the ANA Code of Ethics, that "nursing care is directed toward meeting the comprehensive needs of patients and their families across the continuum of care," it seems clear that nurses have a role in helping dying patients address these obstacles to their emotional, social, and spiritual well-being, as well as providing physical care at the end of life. When dying patients are anguished or suffering emotionally, nurses should encourage them to discuss these crises and explore with them the actions they can take to resolve them. With the patient's permission, for instance, a nurse could contact an estranged family member and explain the situation and the significance of a visit to the patient, to aid a reconciliation that will help the patient achieve a more peaceful death.

The nurse in Case 76 should provide support to this dying patient and his family, but there are limits to what she should do. Clearly she should not deceive the patient's family or participate in any way in the patient's deception by telling them that he has cancer or providing a phony answer to explain why he is not receiving chemotherapy. She must make it evident to the patient that she will not lie for him, though she, of course, will respect the confidentiality of information about his health.

Once the patient has decided to be truthful with his family, there are several ways the nurse can help. She may be able to obtain written materials to help him explain his illness and could help him contact community support agencies or informal groups where a gay patient can get advice and help. She could also offer to meet with him and his family to provide emotional support when he reveals the true nature of his illness. She can be expected to take these steps to help a patient with unfinished business. Any additional efforts would be above and beyond what is morally required.

Case 77

I've become really close to one of my patients who has ALS. We talk about death and what he wants to happen when he can't survive without a ventilator. He has made it clear that he will refuse all treatment before he reaches that point so that he can die peacefully at home. He currently has a feeding tube and we're hydrating him, but he just told me that he is going to start refusing the nutrition. I feel guilty about this because I don't want to stop feeding him, even though prolonging his life is prolonging his misery. **Do I have a responsibility to help him have the kind of death he wants?**

This patient has reached a decision to refuse nutrition in order to die peacefully at home without the use of life-prolonging interventions. This is consistent with the values he identified when he stated that he would refuse a ventilator and any treatment requiring hospitalization at the end of life. Based on the ethical guidelines for the care of dying patients, as established by the ANA Code of Ethics, nurses should provide care in a way that maximizes the values that the dying patient treasures. The nurse should therefore support the patient's decision to refuse nutrition and thereby help him to have the kind of death he has chosen.

Often nurses are uncomfortable when nutrition is withdrawn, especially when the patient has a feeding tube that is left in place, and they may find it frustrating to be unable to provide the usual care for a patient. This would not justify withdrawal from this case, nevertheless, and it would not support any attempt to interfere with the patient's determination that this care be withheld.

However, when a nurse believes that it is wrong to participate in treatment withdrawals designed to bring about death, the nurse has the moral right to seek to transfer the patient's care to another nurse on the grounds of her moral objection. The agency's ethics committee could be consulted for advice in identifying ethically acceptable options for nurses who object to a patient's treatment decisions.

Case 78

Patients who are really sick sometimes think about suicide; sometimes they tell me they want it all to be over, and I know what they mean. I have an AIDS patient, a man who doesn't have a soul in the world except his dog. From the questions he's been asking me lately, I think he wants to know how to end his life without any pain. **What should I do about this?**

The nurse must decide what information she can ethically provide to a patient who may be contemplating suicide and what actions she should take in response. Her first responsibility is to initiate a discussion with the patient to explore his state of mind. If he exhibits severe depression or distorted thinking, the nurse should refer the patient for appropriate counseling. On the other hand, the patient may be a competent man who is seeking to minimize his suffering and maintain some control over the dying process. It is even possible that suicide is rational in certain situations. A nurse would face a serious ethical dilemma if she believed a patient was making a rational choice, torn between the obligation to protect patient confidentiality and the legal requirement to alert others to a potential suicide.

If depression and mental illness have been carefully excluded as the source of the patient's possibly suicidal thoughts, the issue is whether the nurse should answer questions about how to end life without pain. Given the recent publicity about the pros and cons of physician-assisted suicide, a patient may initiate a discussion of assistance in dying.

In Oregon, the only state thus far to have legalized assisted suicide, the Oregon Nurses Association has issued a set of guidelines outlining the nurse's role related to the Death with Dignity Act. Nurses who choose under Oregon's law to participate in assisted suicide may do any of the following:

- Provide care and comfort to the patient and family through all stages of the dying process, as well as teach the patient and family about the process and what to expect.
- Maintain confidentiality concerning the end-of-life decision the patient and family make.
- Explore options with the patient and family regarding end-of-life decisions and provide information that would enable access to available resources.

- Discuss and explore the reasons for the patient's decision in order to determine whether the decision is a result of a depressive illness that would preclude rational decision making.
- Be present during the patient's self-administration of the medication and during the patient's death to ease the family's suffering and provide counsel; and
- Be involved in policy development within the health care facility or community.

Nurses who choose to participate in assisted suicide may not do any of the following:

- Inject or administer the medication that will lead to the death of the patient (This would constitute active euthanasia, which is illegal.)
- Breach confidentiality of patients asking for information about or choosing assisted suicide.
- Make judgmental comments or act with prejudice in response to a patient's questions or choice of assisted suicide.
- Subject peers or other health care professionals to unwarranted, judgmental comments or behavior in reaction to their decision to support and care for a patient who chooses assisted suicide.
- Abandon or refuse to provide palliative care and safety measures to the patient.

Those who choose not to be involved in assisted suicide have corresponding responsibilities to maintain confidentiality, refrain from judgmental comments and acts, provide ongoing care related to comfort and safety measures, and comply with the law governing assisted suicide. In addition, they have the right to conscientiously object to being involved in the care of a patient who chooses suicide. The nurse must transfer care to another provider under the circumstances and may withdraw from the case only when alternative sources of care have been put in place. Nurses who oppose assisted suicide on moral grounds have the same right as those who support it to be involved in policy development within agencies and the community alike.

A patient who asks about assisted suicide presents a good opportunity for a nurse to explore the patient's mental state, his perception of his illness and prognosis, his attitudes toward death and dying, and related topics that reveal the value commitments of the patient. Patients' questions may signal the need for increased pain medications, closer consultation with the physician, referral to a social worker, psychiatric counselor, or religious advisor, or honest conversations between the patient and family. When patients ask questions about dying, nurses have the important responsibility to listen to the concerns that families often dismiss or deny.

ANALYSIS OF CASE 65

Case 65 involves a patient with end-stage cancer who has decided he wants to refuse further treatment and resuscitation. His sons are upset and may try to ignore his wishes if he becomes incompetent. The ethical issue for the nurse is what to do if the patient's sons attempt to have him resuscitated.

Competent patients can exercise their rights to self-determination by completing an advance directive, such as a living will, which expresses their wishes about treatments to be provided when they are terminally ill and incompetent, or a durable power of attorney for health care, which names an agent to make health care decisions for them when they are incompetent. Comfort One bracelets, standard hospital bracelets with Allow Natural Death or Do Not Resuscitate printed on them, authorize emergency medical personnel to carry out an AND or DNR order in the home setting.

As a competent individual, this patient has the right to refuse any life-saving measures. To promote his right to make that decision, the nurse should engage the patient in a discussion of his wishes. She can provide information about advance directives, emphasizing that these documents must be executed while he is fully competent, before either the illness or pain medication puts his judgment in question. If he decides to complete an advance directive, he should be encouraged to provide copies to his sons as well as his physician. He should discuss his wishes with his sons and make sure they understand that this document is legally binding. In addition, he should arrange to obtain a Comfort One bracelet, which would allow paramedics to observe his wishes about resuscitation.

His sons should be informed that, even if there is no advance directive, a surrogate decision maker should use information about the patient's wishes regarding end-of-life treatment to make a decision on the basis of the substituted judgment standard. Absent an advance directive and reliable information about a patient's wishes, a surrogate decision maker must use the best interest or "reasonable person" standard, choosing as a reasonable person would be expected to choose. The reasonable person standard could also support a decision to forgo resuscitation.

Clearly the patient's sons would be wrong to attempt to impose resuscitation on him when he is no longer able to make the decision to reject treatment. If they do attempt to override his wishes, the nurse should intervene to support the patient's wish to forgo resuscitation. She should contact his physician for a DNR order, if that is necessary.

Encouraging a family discussion of these matters should foster a better relationship between father and sons. His sons would be able to voice their concerns and hopefully achieve an understanding of their father's reasons for refusing resuscitation. The nurse should also discuss the services a hospice program could provide, since its philosophy is consistent with the patient's wish to refuse life-saving treatment. Hospice staff has expertise in providing palliative care and can provide emotional support for the patient and his sons.

ETHICAL CRITERIA

- Competent adults always have the right to refuse treatment.
- There is no obligation to provide futile treatment.
- There is no moral difference between withholding and withdrawing treatment.
- Decisions to refuse treatment may be made for incompetent patients.

PRACTICAL STRATEGIES

When a dying patient refuses treatment:

- Determine that the patient's decision is free from coercion.
- Advocate for the patient's right to make the decision.

- Educate the family about the patient's right to refuse treatment.
- Provide the patient with information on hospice care.

When a dying patient has an advance directive:

- Obtain the document for the patient's record.
- Explain to the family what advance directives mean for the patient's care.
- Facilitate effective communication regarding the patient's wishes.
- Champion the rights of the patient when families disagree.

When an incompetent patient has no advance directive:

- Determine whether there is any evidence of the patient's wishes.
- Support the decision the patient would have made, if there is evidence of the patient's wishes.
- Encourage the surrogate decision maker to choose as a reasonableperson would, if there is no evidence of the patient's wishes.

When an incompetent patient's family wants to "do everything":

- Ensure that the family understands the medical facts.
- Explain that there is no moral obligation to provide futile care.

When end-of-life decisions must be made for a dying child:

- Advocate for the best interest of the patient.
- Support the family
- Inform the family about available resources.

If a dying patient is making treatment decisions to protect the family:

- Assess whether this is a competent, informed decision.
- Encourage discussion with the family.
- Respect the patient's decision.

If a dying patient's denial will harm significant others:

- Encourage the patient to accept information about the course of the illness.
- Discuss with the patient the effect of the illness on the family.
- Suggest ways for the family to interact while the patient seeks treatment.
- Provide the family with information regarding support services.

When families disagree with a patent's decision to reject life-sustaining treatment:

- Encourage the patient to discuss the decision with the family.
- Educate the patient's family about the patient's right to refuse treatment.
- Explain the distinction between treatment refusal and suicide.
- Identify support services for the patient and family.

When family members disagree about end-of-life decisions for an incompetent patient:

- Determine who is the patient's surrogate decision maker.
- Arrange a family conference to encourage shared decision making.
- Assist the family in coping with the implications of their decision.

When patients ask for help in taking care of unfinished business:

- Determine whether the request falls within the scope of the nurse's professional responsibilities.
- Consider whether complying with the request is consistent with the ideal character traits sought.
- Realize it is the nurse's choice to go beyond what is morally and professionally required.

When dying patients seek the nurse's help in achieving a good death by refusing nutrition:

- Respect the patient's right to make the decision.

- Recognize that the patient's right to refuse treatment includes the right to forgo nutrition.
- Show concern and compassion even when there is disagreement withthe patient's decision.
- Seek a transfer if the patient's decision conflicts with personal values.

When a dying patient is contemplating suicide:

- Understand what the law prohibits.
- Assist the patient in securing appropriate psychiatric care.
- Identify the reasons for the decision and try to provide remedies.
- Maintain patient confidentiality within the bounds of the law.
- Encourage dialogue with the family.
- Refuse to participate in or facilitate a patient's suicide.

Chapter 8

NURSES' RESPONSIBILITIES, NURSES' RIGHTS

Nurses who accept the professional and moral responsibility of caring for patients in their own homes may question the limits of that responsibility when they encounter situations where patients request more from them than professional nursing care. Some families may also make demands or create difficult situations that raise the question of the rights nurses have to establish boundaries with patients and families

Case 79

I'm working on a case now where the patient's son is a doctor who is interfering in his mom's care. He overrides the medication orders from her doctor or even tells me to skip doses, and then when I don't do what he wants, he complains to the agency that I'm incompetent. His mother goes along with whatever he says. It's an impossible situation. **Would I be justified in refusing to care for this patient?**

General Issues

- **What are the limits of nurses' responsibilities to patients?**
- **What boundaries do nurses have a right to establish with families?**
- **When is a nurse justified in withdrawing from a case?**
- **What moral and legal rights do home health care nurses have?**

INTRODUCTION

Clearly nurses have weighty responsibilities when they care for patients in the patients' own homes. Indeed, individually, home health care nurses may have even greater responsibilities than nurses who practice in an acute care hospital, for there are important differences in these two settings. The hospital setting generally provides an environment that is structured and strictly controlled by health care professionals. Hospitals can safeguard high standards of cleanliness, maintain consistent schedules for treatments and care, supervise the administration of necessary medications, and generally ensure that the care ordered by a physician is given. In the hospital setting, nurses provide skilled care for patients according to a preestablished routine that is ordinarily implemented without significant interference from families.

In the home setting, however, the whole environment is essentially under the control of the family and patient. Families administer medications, establish the standards of cleanliness, determine schedules, and provide most of the care, which must fit in with the other demands of family life. Because the family has this pivotal role, nurses' concerns about the quality of care a patient receives are much more common and more urgent than would be the case in a hospital setting. Given their moral and legal duty to alert others to these concerns, as well as the obligation to assess the safety of patients who live alone and to determine when physicians should be contacted, home health care nurses have significant responsibilities. Importantly, they face all of these responsibilities essentially on their own. They are, of course, part of a team, as nurses are in hospitals, but other health care professionals are not as immediately available for advice or help with critical decisions when a crisis arises in the home. Moreover, nurses are the only ones in a position to provide a total professional assessment of the situation.

A final difference exists in the fact that the hospital setting is an institutional environment which fosters professional relationships, but when nurses visit a patient's home, some families and patients may presume a more personal connection that extends beyond the traditional nurse-patient relationship. This raises issues about the nature of the morally ideal relationship and the moral and professional rights nurses can claim when confronted with demands or expectations that exceed their professional responsibilities or that infringe upon personal or moral boundaries.

THE LIMITS OF NURSES' RESPONSIBILITIES TO PATIENTS

Case 80

I'm caring for a patient who lost her significant other to cancer only three months ago, after a prolonged and very difficult dying process. Soon after her partner died, the patient was diagnosed with cancer herself. She gets chemotherapy and was admitted to our service for the intravenous therapy she needs after the chemo. She lives alone and she is so scared. I've tried to get her to see a counselor, but she refuses because they haven't helped her in the past. She hates her doctor and hates the nurse at the hospital. Apparently I'm the only one she doesn't hate. Lately she's really clinging to me. I see her every two weeks, but she calls me every day. I'm not comfortable at all with this. I want some boundaries. **What limits do I have a right to establish with this patient?**

The notion of setting limits to the relationship a nurse has established with a patient may seem to violate the fundamental ideals of nursing as a caring profession. Most nurses deem caring to be the essence of nursing. According to one prominent nursing scholar this care orientation distinguishes nursing practice from other health care professions that are oriented to disease and cure. However, the ideal of a caring relationship between nurse and patient, though important, provides only the barest direction for actual nursing practice. The question in this case, for example, is whether caring for this patient requires unlimited attention to her significant personal and emotional needs.

In an attempt to clarify the concept of caring and articulate the moral foundation of nursing, nursing scholars have identified various responses, attitudes, and behaviors that exemplify caring. Caring for patients, first of all, involves an appropriate emotional response to a patient's needs. As one influential writer observes, caring is motivated by the capacity to be touched by human suffering and springs from a natural sympathy that humans feel for one another. That emotional response of compassion and sensitivity to a patient's needs has been identified by most nurses as an integral part of caring. This is what "caring for" someone involves, and it is in this sense that caring is said to be an inextricable part of the role of nurses. A good nurse, then, is someone who responds compassionately, who genuinely cares for patients, as opposed to someone who simply carries out the obligatory activities identified in a plan of care with no emotional sensitivity or responsiveness to patient needs.

Second, a good nurse will be motivated to provide nursing services to address the health care needs of patients. Caring in this second sense identifies nursing's primary function, according to one prominent scholar: "Caring is the highest form of commitment to patients." Caring thus involves an attitude toward patients that focuses careful attention on the suffering and needs of patients, with a motivation to use nursing skills to relieve suffering and promote health and healing. This commitment to patients is interpreted by some as patient advocacy, which is said to encompass several nursing activities, such as securing medical intervention when needed, managing patient services from various health care providers, and advocating for care for the whole patient, including attention to the significance of illness in a patient's life.

Third, as other scholars have emphasized, caring for patients means competently utilizing nursing knowledge and nursing skills to address the health care needs of patients. The specific activities that constitute nursing services are thus also part of the concept of caring for patients. Caring in all of these senses is essential to meet the ideal of good nursing practice.

Fourth, and most important, caring is said to define an ethical standard for nursing actions. One nursing scholar states that caring provides "the moral stance from which one intervenes as a nurse." This could be interpreted to mean that caring is also a moral attitude toward patients, a view generally accepted by nurses. However, even this identification of caring with a moral stance does still not offer any specific guidelines for actions and practices in a particular case.

Other theorists identify what is known as an "ethics of care," which recognizes caring as the essential guideline for making moral decisions. The ethics of care emphasizes what some have called women's moral voice of care, a voice of nurturing and concern for other people, their relationships, and their suffering. The ethics of care identifies the value of caring, requires emotional response and sensitivity, values and promotes caring relationships, and attends to the particulars of individuals' situations rather than relying on the application of traditional moral principles.

Unfortunately, the ethics of care, like the general appeal to caring as the moral essence of nursing, fails to provide specific guidance when ethical decisions must be made to resolve a question of the requirements and limits of caring itself. The consensus is that caring is necessary for the ethical practice of nursing, but whether caring is explained as a concern about relieving suffering, an ethical commitment to patients, providing competent nursing care, a moral stance, or a standard for making moral choices, the concept of caring is too vague to provide a sufficient guideline for making moral decisions. Nurses must also be guided by traditional consideration of rights and consequences, and, moving beyond merely traditional considerations, they must pay attention to the particular features of a situation, the ideal of preserving valued relationships, and the goal of developing their own desirable character traits.

Acknowledging all of these considerations is crucial when nurses face issues about setting limits with patients, as in Case 80. The nurse in that case embodies the ideal of caring: she responds with compassion and sensitivity to the needs of this patient; she is motivated to use her nursing skills to alleviate the patient's suffering and attend to her health needs; and she has, it appears, used her skills competently. The question that remains, though, is whether caring requires an unlimited response to the needs and demands of a lonely and despairing woman. If caring is not an unlimited obligation, there must be a justification for establishing appropriate boundaries.

Thus, in addition to the guiding concepts of the ethics of care, ethical nursing practice requires careful reflection on the essential moral factors of rights and consequences, for these factors provide the ethical basis for establishing limits to the obligation of caring for others. Most importantly, caring, in order to be ethical caring, must respect the rights of individuals to make their own decisions based on their ideas of what is valuable and to live their lives according to those ideas. Individuals involved in relationships should not be coerced or manipulated to sacrifice their autonomy or significant personal values in order to maintain the bond. Therefore, though a nurse commits to establishing a caring relationship with a patient, she retains several rights that define the limits of that relationship. One important right relevant to Case 80 is the right to reject intrusive demands on her own personal time, which, based on autonomy, she should be able to use as she chooses.

A careful consideration of the consequences of a nurse-patient relationship without boundaries also provides the basis for establishing limits. A nurse must set limits with an individual patient who demands excessive time and attention. Otherwise, she may be forced to neglect other patients or other professional responsibilities. For example, she may find it difficult to keep her schedule of appointments and she may be unable to give sufficient attention to the health needs of other patients. Given these consequences, the ideal of limitless caring is morally problematic. Limits can be ethically established to allow adequate attention to each patient and also recognize a nurse's right to restrict intrusive demands on her own time.

Though the nurse in this case is justified in establishing these limits, as a caring professional, she should address the fact that this patient says that she hates all the other health care professionals involved in her care, with the result that she has no other emotionally supportive relationships. The nurse should strive to maintain a relationship in which she can provide support for this patient. Other professionals, such as a social worker, could become involved to help address this patient's significant needs.

Case 81

I have a patient who has been on the service for at least a year. Caring for her is one of the biggest challenges I have. She has multiple medical problems, including hypertension and diabetes. I see her twice a week to prefill her insulin which she keeps in a cooler because she doesn't have a refrigerator. Some days she doesn't take her insulin because she's not in the mood. The place is disgusting, trash everywhere. I don't even take my bag into the home because there's no clean place to put it. There's no place for me to sit because the chairs are piled high with old newspapers, so she tells me to sit on the commode. The latest problem is that she is convinced she has an ear infection, but she doesn't have any symptoms. She is insisting that I should tell her doctor she has an ear infection so she can get antibiotics. When I told her I can't do that, she got very angry and abusive. **How far do I have to go to meet my obligations to this patient?**

Caring for patients, the primary function of nursing is a professional commitment to using nursing skills to meet patients' health care needs. The American Nurses Association Code of Ethics articulates the requirement that nurses should deliver nursing services "with respect for human needs and values." The question raised by Case 81 is what that commitment involves in a particular situation. Is caring for patients to be understood as requiring nurses to meet their health care needs as patients identify them? Do nurses have a responsibility to fulfill patients' demands for nursing care? Some patients may expect nurses to facilitate access to treatments they believe they need or to grant a desire for additional nursing services they would like to have, despite a nurse's professional judgment that this is unnecessary. Clearly, the nurse's primary commitment to the patient does not entail an unlimited responsibility to meet such patient demands for nursing care and services, and, for both moral and legal reasons, nurses must refuse any demands that are not warranted based on their professional judgment. The ANA Code of Ethics explicitly recognizes that nurses are justified in refusing to participate in providing services that are inappropriate for a specific patient on the grounds of preserving integrity.

To meet her obligations to this patient, the nurse must of course contact the patient's physician in the event that her assessment does reveal any evidence of a health problem. In addition, as in any case where patients do not "follow orders," she should renew her efforts at educating the patient about the risks she incurs when she does not take her insulin. She may also refer the patient for counseling and other services, and should inform the patient's physician, as well as her nursing supervisor, of this situation.

This patient also challenges the nurse's ability to fulfill the ethical commitment to provide care without prejudice. According to the ANA Code of Ethics, "A fundamental principle that underlies all nursing practice is respect for the inherent worth, dignity, and human rights of every individual." The nurse should deliver nursing services "unrestricted by considerations of social or economic status, personal attributes, or the nature of health problems."

The reality of home health care is that this ideal is frequently challenged, perhaps more significantly than is the case in other settings in which nurses practice. Home health care patients sometimes have multiple medical problems that make them difficult to care for successfully at home, or their families or other caregivers may interfere with proper care. Other patients live in dangerous neighborhoods, maintain very dirty homes, or choose lifestyles that are offensive to many nurses. Moreover, some individuals are personally hostile, uncooperative, and disrespectful. Because of such personal characteristics, which can be exaggerated in the home setting and thus difficult to ignore, some patients are what references in the literature refer to as "the hateful patient," a patient with whom it may seem virtually impossible to form a caring relationship. Nurses may experience intense feelings and personal reactions when they confront these realities which seem to threaten their ability to meet the professional and moral ideal of providing care without prejudice.

Certainly there is a sense in which individuals cannot control such natural feelings, but this fact of human nature is not an insurmountable obstacle to establishing a caring relationship with a patient. Good nurses will respond compassionately and with sensitivity to the needs of even "hateful patients" and thereby succeed in creating a caring relationship. Finally, an essential aspect of a caring relationship is that care be delivered in a certain way. Caring in this sense refers to the professional actions nurses perform in providing nursing services, rather than simply the personal feelings a nurse has about a particular patient. Caring involves treating patients with respect and without prejudice and respecting their rights as patients, regardless of those personal feelings.

Case 82

> I had a private pay patient, a man my age who had broken his hip. We really hit it off. He was immobile in the beginning but by the end of the second week, he didn't really need skilled nursing care. I was basically getting paid to hang out with him. He actually made up a schedule for nursing visits and expected me to fill all of it. He called and asked the agency to cancel all of my other patients and send me there. The agency agreed to do that. I told them he doesn't need me, he just wants a friend, but the agency assigned me to his case. **What right do I have to refuse an assignment I consider unprofessional?**

In effect, this patient wants to maintain his relationship with the nurse when there is no professional basis for a continuing relationship, that is, he no longer has health needs that require skilled nursing care. He is presuming that the relationship is a personal one that he can choose to pursue. This raises an issue about the ethically appropriate limits of the nurse-patient relationship and the extent of the nurse's commitment to care for the patient. Nurses, according to the International Council of Nurses, have four fundamental responsibilities: "to promote health, to prevent illness, to restore health and to alleviate suffering." Given that this is the foundation of the nurse-patient relationship, nurses have the responsibility to recognize and maintain the boundaries that are thereby established, as the ANA Code states. Thus, the responsibilities nurses have to care for patients and to advocate for patients are limited to professional activities that contribute to the patient's health.

Nonetheless, since nursing care involves personal contact with patients, some individuals may expect nurses to assent to a more intimate relationship than the professional boundaries permit, especially when nurses provide care in the patient's own home. Similarly, some patients or families may want to show their appreciation to nurses with substantial gifts or invitations to be involved in family celebrations, or propose other shared activities. Given that maintaining a professional nurse-patient relationship is the moral ideal, nurses have the responsibility to clearly identify the limits of the relationship. Substantial gifts as well as attempts to engage nurses in inappropriate personal connections must therefore be refused. This nurse is justified in refusing to allow a personal friendship, since that would violate professional boundaries.

Moreover, nurses have the right to object to the misuse of their time and their professional skills to serve some purpose apart from addressing a patient's health needs. The agency should respect the nurse's professional judgment that this patient does not have a health problem which requires nursing care and refuse the patient demand that she keep the schedule of visits that he has developed. Undoubtedly the agency has violated this nurse's rights by assigning her to care for a patient who has no skilled nursing needs.

Case 83

There is a patient I have been seeing for two months. He is so grateful for the care I have provided that he insists he wants to do something to show his appreciation. He is a financial planner and investment advisor and has offered to make some recommendations for investments, without charging his usual fee. **Should I refuse his offer to do me this favor?**

Accepting financial advice from this patient would constitute a business relationship, an additional association between nurse and patient that lies outside the boundaries of the professional relationship. When nurses and patients also become involved in other roles, these associations should be scrutinized to determine whether the dual relationship is ethically objectionable.

Sometimes nurses cannot avoid being involved in a second relationship in addition to the professional relationship with a patient. If a nurse works and lives in a small community, her next patient may also be a neighbor, a fellow church member, or a familiar figure from community activities. These dual relationships are ordinarily unobjectionable, though they may pose ethical challenges, such as maintaining professional boundaries with a neighbor, respecting the privacy of individuals the nurse knows from other associations, and protecting the confidentiality of medical information.

On the other hand, many dual relationships would violate the professional responsibility to maintain appropriate boundaries with patients. There are also criteria that are useful in deciding when and why a relationship with a patient is ethically wrong. First, the relationship is not in the patient's best interest or, even if it benefits the patient, it primarily serves the nurse's own interest. Second, the relationship is exploitative because it "uses" the patient and the uneven power relationship between the nurse and the patient to benefit the nurse. Third, the relationship introduces a conflict of interest between the actions required in the role of the nurse and the actions necessary as a friend or business partner. Fourth, the dual relationship clouds or distorts the nurse's professional judgment. All of these reasons may be summarized as the recognition that the dual relationship will harm the patient in some way.

In Case 83, entering into a business relationship with the patient would appear to benefit the nurse because she is accepting the gift of valuable financial advice from the patient. This dual relationship exploits the patient, serves the nurse's interest more than the patient's interest, and may present a conflict of interest if the nurse continues to care for him. Therefore, the nurse must refuse the patient's offer of financial and investment advice.

ESTABLISHING BOUNDARIES WITH FAMILIES

Case 84

Sometimes the real problem I have is not the patient but someone in the family. I am caring for a forty-year-old man who is physically incapacitated. His wife does not take very good care of him. She has her own ideas about what he needs and ignores anything she doesn't agree is necessary. Then she orders me to do what she has decided should be done, even things that could be harmful. When I don't do what she wants she is very abusive. **How much do I have to put up with from a patient's family?**

Apart from concerns about the quality of care the family member provides in this case, there are important issues about the boundaries nurses can justifiably establish with families. Though many nurses and families grow close when they share the task of caring for a patient, nurses have the responsibility to maintain professional boundaries with families as well as with the patient and should not allow the relationship with the family to become an inappropriate personal relationship. The limits that should be set are justified by the professional purpose of the nurse-family collaboration.

On the other hand, in some difficult situations the nurse-family relationship is not characterized by emotional closeness but instead by the tension that serious illness causes, conflicts over patient care, or disagreements about the role of the nurse. Some families expect the nurse to simply comply with their "orders" for patient services, disregarding the professional role of the nurse to provide the skilled care ordered by the patient's physician or interfering with the care of the patient. Other family caregivers may direct considerable rage, hostility, or abuse at nurses. These actions violate the basic right that nurses have to be treated with respect as professionals.

When a family member's behavior continues to violate the professional boundaries the nurse has identified, or when the behavior is abusive or restricts the nurse's ability to care for a patient, the nurse has the right to withdraw from the case. Agencies can require patients and families to enter into contracts which specify the rights and responsibilities of both parties. They have the right to terminate the contract if patients or family members fail to meet their responsibilities, as long as they give fair notice and provide the opportunity to find alternative care. In Case 84, the agency could establish a contract with the patient that states that the agency will withdraw if the family continues the abusive treatment of the nurse and interferes with the nurse's care of the patient. The appropriate authorities must also be contacted if the family member's behavior constitutes a serious risk to the well-being of the patient.

At the same time, it is important to consider the patient's family relationships and the consequences any actions the nurse initiates could have for those relationships. Even though the patient is receiving substandard care from his wife, he may prefer to maintain the *status quo* rather than do anything that would anger or upset her. That is a judgment that a competent patient has the right to make, and it ordinarily should be respected. The nurse should attempt to have a private discussion with the patient to ascertain his wishes.

Case 85

One of my patients is a ten-year-old boy who was severely burned on his abdomen and lower extremities when he started a fire playing with matches. I see him several times each week to change his burn dressings. This is a complex, painful, and time-consuming process, which he hates. He continually pinches me while I'm trying to change his dressings; I'm black and blue when I leave there, but his mother won't do anything about it. She's so focused on his injuries that she allows him to do whatever he wants. Several nurses have refused to be involved in his care because of this. If I ask out, too, I'm afraid the agency will want to withdraw from this case. **Am I obligated to tolerate this in order to meet my responsibility to care for this patient?**

When a nurse cares for a child who mistreats her, her first response should be to attempt to establish limits with the parents. If that is not successful and the parents continue to allow the problematic behavior, the nurse should inform her supervisor of the situation. Nurses are not obligated to tolerate mistreatment in order to provide care for a child. It is the responsibility of an agency to make this clear to families by establishing a contract which specifies the responsibilities a family has and clearly states that the agency will withdraw if mistreatment continues.

The conflict for the nurse in this case arises because she believes that her commitment to care for this patient is the primary consideration, despite the mistreatment she suffers. Nonetheless, her responsibility to this child does not require her to ignore her own rights to respectful treatment. Tolerating this kind of mistreatment in order to care for a patient goes above and beyond a nurse's professional and moral duties. She has the right to establish firm boundaries with the child's mother and, if that fails, she would be justified in asking the agency to assign another nurse, even though the result may be that the agency decides to terminate the agreement to care for this child.

WITHDRAWING FROM A CASE

Case 86

I'm often frightened when I go out to patients' homes. Even though we have an escort system we can use if it's a dangerous area, it's not just the bad neighborhoods that frighten me. I have a wealthy patient who lives with his son in one of the best neighborhoods in the city. His son scares me. He makes strange requests, he orders me around, and he is belligerent. I think he's dangerous. **Would I be justified in withdrawing from this case because I think I'm unsafe?**

Though nurses have the responsibility to protect the safety of patients, in some situations, the safety of the nurses themselves is threatened. The Joint Commission on Accreditation of Healthcare Organizations requires home health care agencies to plan for a secure environment and to engage in ongoing training to deal with threats to safety that might arise in the home setting. These include domestic violence, substance abuse, dangerous neighborhoods, and weapons in the home. Many agencies arrange for a member of the police or a security guard to accompany nurses on home visits to dangerous neighborhoods. Based on concerns about staff safety, home health care agencies have a right to refuse to enter into a contract with a potential patient or to withdraw from care if a patient's behavior breaches a contract that has been established.

As part of their professional practice, nurses and other health care professionals must risk some dangers, such as caring for patients with contagious diseases. Yet there are other dangers, like providing care for a threatening patient, that they should not be expected to face if they cannot be sufficiently protected. Nurses are therefore certainly justified in asking to withdraw from cases where they believe they are unsafe, including situations where a member of the patient's family is the source of a nurse's concerns about her safety.

When nurses ask to withdraw, they must fully inform the agency about the behavior or situation that concerns them, so that other nurses assigned to the case have the information they need to decide whether to accept the assignment. Work under such dangerous circumstances should only be on a volunteer basis.

Case 87

I'm seeing a patient who is recovering from injuries suffered in an accident at work. I'm there for wound care three times a week. Every time I see him, he uses vulgar language and makes sexual advances. I have made it clear to him that this is inappropriate and unwelcome behavior, but he just laughs. If I get the case transferred to another nurse, she will face the same harassment, so I've been trying to ignore it. **What are my rights in these circumstances?**

Based on federal law, nurses have a legal right to work in an environment that is free of discrimination and harassment. Since home health care agencies have an explicit responsibility to support the legal rights of the individuals they employ, they should inform patients that sexual advances and vulgar language are illegal and make clear their intention to uphold the law.

From the perspective of this nurse, the more pressing concern is whether she should withdraw from the case, given the likelihood that any female assigned will face the same vulgar remarks and offensive behavior. She has apparently chosen to subject herself to this mistreatment in order to protect other nurses, but this kind of self-sacrifice is unnecessary. She would be justified in requesting to withdraw from the case, based on her right to practice in a setting where she is not subjected to discrimination and harassment. The nurse should report this offensive behavior to her supervisor to ensure that the agency takes the necessary steps to avoid placing another nurse in a situation where she is harassed. The ideal solution would be to assign a male nurse to this case, though he, too, may be subjected to the patient's vulgarity.

Case 88

I have a case where the patient is recovering from a serious head injury. I'm trying to provide the nursing care she needs, but I can't get any cooperation from her, and I don't think anyone else could either. A mental health evaluation found her to be of sound mind so she has the legal right to make the decisions about her care. Even though she is incontinent of both urine and stool, she refuses a Foley catheter, and she has only two pairs of pants to wear, which she never washes. **Exactly what legal rights do I have to withdraw from a case? Would I be risking my license if I back out of this case?**

The key question in Case 88 is the extent of a nurse's legal right to withdraw from a case without endangering her license to practice. A nursing license could be denied, revoked, or suspended if a nurse is guilty of unprofessional conduct. Unprofessional conduct includes, but is not limited to, abandonment of a patient, willfully making and filing false reports in the practice of nursing, failing to file reports as required by law, failing to provide details of a patient's nursing needs to succeeding nurses qualified to care for the patient, willful disregard of the standards of nursing practice, and failure to maintain the standards established by the nursing profession. Under certain circumstances, a nurse who refuses to accept a patient or to continue caring for a patient could be charged with insubordination and abandonment, which is unprofessional conduct, and lose her license.

The Nurse Practice Acts outline the legal boundaries of nursing practice in each state. If charges of abandonment or negligence were to arise, these acts would be used, in part, to determine the standard of care. Each state also has a State Board of Nursing, and their regulations, along with state and federal law, contribute to establishing standards of care, as well. Home health care standards would also be used where relevant to determine if unprofessional conduct has occurred, because determining professional conduct is influenced by the setting for providing care.

Nurses must meet the objective standard of care in order to comply with the laws regarding negligence and avoid malpractice. The standard of care mandates acting as a "reasonable prudent nurse" would act in similar circumstances. Negligent behavior is that which falls below the standard of care. Malpractice is a type of negligence referring to professional responsibilities. A nurse can be found guilty of malpractice if the courts demonstrate: (1) there was a duty the nurse had toward a particular patient, (2) the nurse breached this duty, (3) the patient was injured, and (4) the breach of duty caused the patient's injuries.

The patient in Case 88 is competent and thus has the right to accept or refuse treatment. Her decisions, however, such as her refusal of a catheter, could make it difficult for the nurse to meet the standard of care. The nurse must document this situation to establish her efforts to satisfy the objective standard of care and avoid charges of unprofessional conduct, negligence, or malpractice. As discussed in earlier cases, the agency can establish a contract that sets out the requirements for continuing care. Finally, the nurse can withdraw from the case without the risk of losing her license provided that she follows the procedures outlined in the agency's policies.

MORAL AND LEGAL RIGHTS OF HOME HEALTH CARE NURSES

Case 89

My patient has had three strokes in the last year. Her doctor was so cold and brutal when he talked to her: "I don't see any potential for improvement beyond your present level of functioning. The reality is you won't get any better. You should be in a nursing home." All her therapists disagreed with her doctor, but the agency agreed and pulled everyone out of the home. **What rights do I have when I disagree with the agency's decision to discharge a patient?**

From a legal perspective, nurses are bound by contractual obligations to their employer agencies and to their patients, as well as being legally obligated to follow physicians' orders unless an error has been made or harm may be done to the patient. Apart from these circumstances, nurses appear to have no legal rights to act contrary to physician or agency decisions. From a moral perspective, however, this nurse should advocate with the agency and the physician to attempt to get the patient the services she believes the patient needs in the home setting the patient desires. In a case such as this where the patient's wishes conflict with the decisions of the physician and the agency, the ANA Code of Ethics urges nurses to work to resolve that conflict. Where the conflict is not resolved, the nurse's ethical commitment remains to the patient.

Case 90

Once people are out of the hospital, their doctors don't want to hear about it. There was one lady who had cancer with extensive metastases. I'm surprised she's still alive. I saw her two days after she got out of the hospital. She was not feeling well; she had low blood pressure; she was orthostatic. I called her doctor, but he wouldn't order anything. He said: "How well do you know her? She's a complainer." I argued with him: "Her numbers speak for themselves: 70/40 when she stood up. Take her back and rehydrate her." He wouldn't do it. **What's my responsibility as a patient advocate in this case? What rights do I have when I disagree with the physician's decision?**

The doctor's failure to respond to the patient's low blood pressure may not harm this patient's long-term interest, given her extensive disease and poor prognosis, but the patient could probably be made to feel more comfortable. Though her nurse has advocated with the physician to re-admit the patient in order to address her dehydration, the physician has refused. Do nurses have a responsibility to do anything more in order to secure treatment that may not promote health and healing but could make a patient more comfortable?

Because the necessity of providing this care has been disputed by the physician, there may be little more that a nurse can do from a legal perspective. There is no legal obligation to pursue this further because there is no overt need to protect this patient from the harmful actions of other professionals. However, home health care nurses have the responsibility of providing a nursing assessment of a patient's condition and the moral obligation to take appropriate action based on their professional judgment of the patient's needs. This nurse therefore has the duty to advocate aggressively on behalf of the patient to obtain the care she believes is necessary, and she has the right to express her viewpoint in any appropriate way that she believes will help the patient.

As a professional with the responsibility of providing an assessment of a patient's condition the nurse has a basis for requesting the agency establish a process for addressing such disputes about patient care. She could also ask the agency to consider adopting an appeals process that nurses could use when the dispute with a physician appears to be unsolvable.

Case 91

My patient has lung cancer. The problem is that his physician has not monitored his care closely enough. I told him his nutrition is very poor, but he hasn't addressed it. Now his pain control is inadequate. Today I called his physician to try to get him to see him. He was irate, rude, yelling at me: "If you're such an alarmist, send him to the ER!" He dismissed my assessment out of hand and refused to see him. **What can I do when the doctor disregards my nursing judgment?**

Nurses have a legal responsibility to perform nursing assessments and communicate those assessments to the physician. These professional judgments deserve the respect of other health care professionals, but the reality is that in some cases, physicians may disregard a nurse's evaluation of a patient's health care needs. When a physician dismisses her nursing judgment, as in Case 91, the nurse must assess whether the situation is sufficiently serious to require immediate action on behalf of the patient. As a patient advocate, nurses have the moral, legal, and professional responsibility to respond when the actions of a co-worker or others endanger the patient's welfare. She should raise these issues with her supervisor at her agency and discuss alternatives for getting the patient the care she believes he needs.

On the other hand, nurses and doctors sometimes have genuine disagreements about the care a patient needs. Physicians have the legal authority to determine medical diagnoses and to order treatment that nurses have a duty to carry out, unless they believe there is an error or the possibility of foreseeable harm to the patient. If a nurse carries out an order that has an error or that harms a patient, she may be legally responsible for the harm that results. Nurses consequently have the legal responsibility to assess a doctor's orders and to seek clarification of any orders that seem questionable. Decisions to refuse to carry out physicians' orders should be fully documented. It is also important to document the events when a physician rejects a nurse's assessment of a patient's condition. If a physician or hospital were sued for malpractice, the question of whether the nurse kept the physician informed could be a central issue.

Case 92

I don't want to be involved at all when patients or families decide to stop treatment at the end of life because I think it's wrong for anyone to do anything that might hasten death. That's why it's really a dilemma for me when the doctor writes an order to stop tube feedings for a dying patient. **Do I have a right to refuse to care for patients who are not being fed?**

From a moral perspective, all individuals have the right to make decisions and plan their lives on the basis of their own ideas and values, without coercion from others. This important right to self-determination is jeopardized for any nurse who is required to participate in treatment she thinks is morally wrong. Based on self-determination, then, this nurse has the right to refuse to care for patients who are not being fed. Moreover, this right is recognized in the ANA Code of Ethics which explicitly states that nurses have a responsibility to preserve their own integrity. This comprises an obligation to act consistently with their personal and professional values. If a practice is morally objectionable, as in this case, the nurse is justified in refusing to participate on moral grounds. The ANA Code identifies the conditions for refusing participation: "The nurse is obliged to provide for the patient's safety, to avoid patient abandonment, and to withdraw only when assured that alternative sources of nursing care are available to the patient." Still, depending on the jurisdiction and circumstances, nurses may not be protected from termination of employment or other sanctions if they in fact refuse to provide care on the grounds of conscience.

This kind of situation evokes what one philosopher defines as moral distress, the anguish that arises when a nurse believes that she is prevented from doing what is morally right, by institutional constraints, for instance, and she feels compelled to act against her own judgment about what is right to do. In short, nurses suffer moral distress when they feel their integrity is in jeopardy.

An important source of moral distress, as one author claims, are situations such as Case 92 where nurses are compelled to participate in actions that violate their own personal beliefs. One study of moral distress among nurses working in a hospital setting identified three additional factors in nurses' moral distress: situations where a nurse has knowledge of a patient's needs and values and, as a consequence, disagrees with the care supported by the family or by the policies of the health care institution; circumstances where the nurse believes that the actions being undertaken are not to the benefit of the patient; and, finally, situations that involve deception. When nurses' professional goals are blocked and nurses are not able to fulfill their commitment to a patient, scholars agree, nurses experience moral distress.

Because moral distress has often been found to be a major factor in burnout among nurses, home health care agencies, as well as hospitals, should provide access to an agency ethics committee or an equivalent process which can address moral conflicts between nurses and physicians, as well as provide a forum for voicing questions concerning the ethical aspects of nursing practice and acquiring advice and support from other nurses. Studies have also underscored the significance of an ethical decision-making model in helping nurses address moral conflicts and thereby reduce the stress of such situations.

Some agencies may limit services according to moral ideals, which are often based on religious values. A nurse who feels strongly about the kinds of services she is willing to provide could seek employment with an agency that shares her values or at least seek an agreement to avoid assignment to certain kinds of cases.

Home health care nurses have the legal, professional, and moral responsibility to promote and protect patients' health, safety, and rights. Nurses also have rights arising from their professional role in providing competent nursing care, in addition to the rights all individuals have based on widely accepted moral standards, such as the right to work in an environment that is safe and free of discrimination and harassment. The American Nurses Association's Bill of Rights for Registered Nurses recognizes nurses' rights to practice in a setting that enables them to meet professional standards and supports ethical practice. In addition, nurses have the right to withdraw from a case under certain circumstances, such as situations where they believe a practice is morally objectionable.

ANALYSIS OF CASE 79

Case 79 describes a situation where the patient's son, a doctor, is interfering in his mom's care and overriding medication orders. When the nurse does not comply with his orders, he complains to the agency that she is incompetent. The ethical issue is whether the nurse would be justified in refusing to care for this patient.

This situation evokes fundamental questions about the extent of the responsibilities nurses have to patients and families and the moral and legal rights nurses can claim. Nurses' responsibilities have their basis in the nurse's primary commitment to the health, safety, and rights of the patient. The nurse's most important duty in Case 79 is to advocate on behalf of the patient's health and safety, since the patient may be harmed by the actions of her son when he insists that medication dosages be skipped or medication orders changed. The potential consequences of allowing this situation to continue unchallenged thus justify a decision to seek intervention from the patient's physician or the home health care agency. Moreover, if the nurse believes that there is a serious threat to the patient's well-being, she has a legal obligation to take appropriate action.

This case also raises another question concerning the nurse's legal responsibilities. When the patient's son prevents the nurse from providing the medications ordered by the patient's own doctor, his interference may make it difficult for the nurse to meet the objective standard of care, which could subject this nurse to a charge of negligence or malpractice. Further, she must deal with the moral distress produced when she is prevented from caring for the patient in the way she believes is appropriate. For those reasons, the nurse has the right to object to his interference with the performance of her professional duties. She should document these incidents carefully and report them as necessary to the patient's own physician and to her supervisor.

Though nurses strive to establish a caring relationship with a patient, the involvement with patients and families is justifiably limited by the professional purpose of the relationship and by the professional and moral rights of nurses. The nurse's mistreatment, including the son's unfair complaints of her incompetence, violates her fundamental right to be treated with respect as a professional.

Nurses are undeniably justified in requesting to withdraw from a case where a family member is interfering with their ability to meet their responsibility to care for the patient. The nurse would therefore be justified in refusing to care for this woman, provided she avoids abandoning the patient and withdraws only when other nursing services have been arranged. She should suggest that the agency establish a contract with this patient and family that would outline their rights and responsibilities as a condition for continuing to provide nursing services.

ETHICAL CRITERIA

- Nurses have a responsibility to promote, advocate for, and strive to protect the health, safety, and rights of the patient.
- Nurses have the responsibility to establish professional boundries with patients and family.
- Nurses have the right to set limits with patients and families.
- Nurses have the right to practice in a setting that enables them to meet professional standards.

- Nurses have the right to work in an environment that supports ethical practice.
- Nurses have the right to withdraw from a case under certain circumstances.

PRACTICAL STRATEGIES

When patients' demands exceed the bounds of professional responsibility:

- Determine whether meeting these demands would interfere with professional responsibilities.
- Establish limits with the patient, as needed.
- Refuse requests that conflict with professional and legal standards.

When families interfere with care:

- Discuss the problematic behavior with the family.
- Have the agency establish a contract which outlines expectations concerning conduct.

When a nurse finds the environment distressing or threatening:

- Discuss concerns with the supervisor.
- Enlist the help of a social worker, if possible.
- Have the agency establish a contract to outline the limits of conduct.
- Withdraw from the case as a last resort.

When a nurse disagrees with a physician's orders or the agency's decisions:

- Advocate for getting the patient the needed care.
- Discuss with the supervisor.
- Consult the agency ethics committee.

When a nurse cannot in good conscience do what is asked:

- Contact the supervisor.
- Request that another nurse take over the care of the patient.

Chapter 9

CARING FOR THE MENTALLY ILL

The effect a patient's illness has on other people may be a cause for special concern when patients have been diagnosed with a mental illness. These concerns must be weighed against the nurse's primary responsibility to promote health and protect the rights of these vulnerable patients.

Case 93

The landlords take care of so many of these patients who live alone. I have an elderly patient with dementia who is hallucinating. Last week he thought the place was burning down. He was knocking on people's doors in the middle of the night and trying to drag them out of their apartments. His landlord called me the next day to say: "Isn't this man a patient of yours? You better do something. He shouldn't be living alone." **What rights does a patient have in these circumstances?**

General Issues

- **What rights do mental health patients have?**
- **What is the patient advocacy role of the psychiatric nurse?**
- **What special responsibilities do nurses have when patients have a diagnosis of mental illness?**
- **When is mandatory treatment justified?**

INTRODUCTION

Nurses generally are assigned to care for mental health patients who reside in the community when they suffer from a persistent, severe mental illness, or they have both a mental health problem and another medical problem. In this setting, psychiatric nursing care usually focuses on managing medications, which are frequently prescribed for use on an "as needed" basis, and evaluating the need for hospitalization for treatment. Because the mental health patient's environment is often a critical factor for successful treatment, the differences that exist between the hospital setting and the patient's own home can be consequential. In the less restrictive setting of the home, patients are more vulnerable to various factors that may affect their health or safety. The patient's home environment may be chaotic, stressful, or violent, with patients sometimes dependent on family caregivers who deny the need for treatment or interfere with medication schedules and treatment plans. Where families have played a role in the development of the patient's mental health problem, if the patient suffered abuse or violence, for example, the patient's illness may worsen due to more frequent contact with family members than they would have in a hospital setting. If an exacerbation of a patient's symptoms occurs, nurses have the responsibility to assess whether a crisis exists and notify a physician or the proper authorities.

Nurses also have the responsibility to advocate for patient rights which may conflict with the rights and interests of others, since the behaviors of mental health patients are sometimes offensive, disturbing, or even threatening to other people. When mental health patients are hospitalized, the effects of their behaviors are limited in a significant way because they are isolated from the community. Patients who are dangerous to self or to others can be carefully monitored and, if necessary, placed in a locked inpatient unit. Additional measures can be taken to restrict a patient's contact with others and impose substantial control over patient behavior. Patients living in the community, however, are subject to minimal restrictions on their behavior. Nurses may have to weigh concerns about other people against the commitment to the patient, a responsibility that seldom arises in the same way when patients are hospitalized and nurses can focus almost exclusively on the needs of the patient. Moreover, home health care nurses have significant concerns about their moral and legal responsibilities when their mental health patients are vulnerable to exploitation or mistreatment, demonstrate impaired judgment, or threaten the safety and welfare of others.

RIGHTS OF MENTAL HEALTH PATIENTS

Case 94

I'm always concerned about the safety of my patients. I have a young patient who lives on the third floor of an old house. This is a good apartment for him. He can't tolerate public housing because he can't stand to have people around him. The problem is that there is a crack house on the first floor. When he comes home, there are usually a couple of addicts hanging around sitting on the front steps. They ask him to pay money to get into his apartment, and he pays. I'm worried that this will escalate, but he prefers to put up with it. He doesn't want me to call the police. **Should I do something about this, even though he disagrees?**

The question is whether the nurse should intervene in order to protect the safety and well-being of a mental health patient against his wishes. This may seem like the right thing to do. Given their greater vulnerability to mistreatment and exploitation by other people, these patients often appear to need nurses and families to intervene in their lives for their own good. However, unless a mental health patient is incompetent or makes decisions that are uninformed or involuntary, such paternalism cannot be justified. As is true for competent patients generally, mentally ill patients who are competent have the moral and legal right to make their own decisions about where they will live and the risks they are willing to take. This patient's decision to acquiesce to requests for money is apparently voluntary and informed, and there is no evidence that he has been explicitly threatened or that he has been physically coerced into making that decision. The nurse can appropriately use persuasion and education, and she should monitor the situation to assure herself that he has not been forced to agree to these requests. But as long as he continues knowingly and willingly to prefer this living situation over his other options, she should not intervene.

It is important to note that remaining in a housing situation that is not safe does not necessarily signify incompetence. Even mentally ill individuals who choose to live on the streets are not, on that basis, considered incompetent. Many patients, indeed, report that they feel safer on the streets than in shelters or institutions. Thus, remaining on the streets or deciding to live in unsafe housing should not be regarded as sufficient to warrant paternalistic intervention.

This case also raises questions about the responsibilities nurses have when patients report illegal behavior. If the nurse has evidence that illegal drug activity is taking place in this house, she faces a dilemma about her responsibilities to public health and safety, which appear to conflict with her obligation to respect a patient's wishes.

Case 95

I have a patient who is a schizophrenic. Now he is hearing voices, so his psychiatrist prescribed a new medication. His wife told me: "He won't take this if he knows it's for the voices." **Should I volunteer the information if he doesn't ask?**

Concern that mental health patients who need medications will refuse to take them appears to justify withholding information in order to get them to cooperate in their treatment. Nonetheless, patients who are competent have the right to give or withhold informed consent to any treatment, including medications for mental health problems. They can only exercise valid consent, however, with adequate and truthful disclosure of the treatment options, together with the risks and benefits of each option. This information, together with any other information that is relevant to a treatment decision, must be provided in a way that is responsive to the needs of the patient. The fact that patients may be cognitively impaired, suffering from mental illness, or diagnosed with a substance abuse problem may complicate communication, but nurses and physicians must provide appropriate information. Patients should not in any case be deceived about the medications they are receiving, no matter how great the risk is that they will refuse to take them.

This nurse should therefore fully inform the patient about his new medication, whether or not he specifically asks what the drug is. Perhaps he will consent to take this new drug if he is educated further about the reasons for the change in medications and the goals of this treatment. Still, as long as he is competent, he has the right to refuse this medication as well as any other treatment for his schizophrenia unless treatment has been mandated by a court order.

Informed consent to treatment is usually explicit. In some cases, though, patients give their implicit or implied consent simply by being cooperative. This, too, constitutes valid consent. Patients also give their implied consent in situations where they make no objection to a procedure when the nurse asks permission or when she prepares to begin a procedure. In the latter case, especially with patients whose psychological or cognitive limitations make them vulnerable, nurses must be sure patients know that they can object if they wish.

Case 96

I had a referral for an assessment of a patient's mental health status. His private duty nurse met me at the door. She said: "Can you see him but not tell him why you're here? I think it might upset him." **Would it be wrong to assess his mental health first, then decide what to tell him?**

Given this patient's vulnerability and his unknown mental health status, the nurse may conclude she should agree in order to avoid upsetting him. This is the claim of therapeutic privilege, the idea that withholding information is justified because disclosure would hinder treatment, pose a risk of psychological damage to the patient, or render the patient incapable of making a rational decision. This may be thought to justify the assessment of a patient's mental health without obtaining informed consent. The claim of therapeutic privilege, though, should always be scrutinized carefully. Only convincing evidence of a clear risk of such harm would justify the failure to disclose the purpose of an assessment and the failure to seek informed consent.

Moreover, a patient should not be assumed to lack the capacity to consent to a mental health evaluation. Though an individual may not be competent in a particular area, such as financial matters, he or she might still be competent to make decisions about medical treatments. Hence, a patient's capacity to make a particular medical decision should be assessed independently of his or her competence to make other choices at the time a decision is required.

In this case, it would be wrong to assess this patient's mental health without his permission. As a competent patient, he should be asked to give his informed consent, which he cannot do if he lacks the relevant information about the purpose of the nurse's visit. His cooperation with an assessment cannot be construed as implicit consent, either, if this information is withheld. Assessing the mental health status of patients without consent can only be justified if there is evidence that the patient is so severely impaired that he or she does not have the capacity to give informed consent for any treatment or evaluation. In that event, permission should be sought from a surrogate decision maker.

Case 97

> I have a male patient in his early twenties who is living with his parents. He suffers from a major mental illness. His mother understands that he needs help, but his father doesn't believe there is anything wrong with him. He doesn't believe his son should be on medications. His father told him: "You're not going to take this." Then he told me: "He doesn't need this. He'll snap out of it if you just leave him alone." **What role should his family have in these decisions?**

Even when mental health patients are competent and should be allowed to make their own decisions without interference, families often try to make treatment decisions for them. Clearly, nurses must support the competent patient's right to decide when families attempt to interfere. At the same time, this nurse can encourage the family to discuss together the options the patient has and their concerns about his treatment and his illness. Patients and families could use shared decision-making processes when decisions about care and treatment must be made that will affect all of them. The final decision, nevertheless, remains with a competent patient. This patient should be the one to decide whether he takes medication for his illness. His father should not be allowed to veto his son's decisions.

The father's comments reveal that he may not accept the general theory of mental illness that governs the treatment for his son. The prevailing medical model holds that many, if not all, mental health problems have a biological basis or cause. According to this model, mental illness is parallel to physical illness and should be treated in similar ways. Psychotropic drugs are thus seen as appropriate and effective methods for treating such illnesses. Instead of accepting the idea that mental illness has a biological basis, though, some people view mental illness as a kind of moral failing that can be controlled by effort and willpower. Medications are sometimes considered unnecessary or a sign of moral weakness. This is apparently the view of the patient's father who thinks his son can "snap out of it."

In response, the nurse should increase her efforts to educate the patient's family about his illness and the need for psychiatric medications. She might also recommend that a social worker or counselor get involved to help the family address the conflicts created by the patient's mental health problem. Ultimately, if the patient's father attempts to prevent his son from taking the prescribed medications, it may be necessary to report this to the appropriate authorities.

Case 98

There are a lot of family issues with mental health patients. I have a twenty-two-year-old patient who is living with his parents. They were giving him his medications for a while, then they stopped because of the side effects. As a result, he became disruptive, pacing at night, swearing at his father, and washing his hands obsessively. They started his medications again for a few days, but now his parents have decided they don't want him on any medication. It turns out that they are philosophically opposed to medicating patients for mental illness. They asked me to help them get him committed to a psychiatric facility. **What should I do if I disagree with his family about what is the best treatment for him?**

It is important, first, to determine whether this patient chose to stop taking his medications, which, of course, is his right. On the other hand, if his parents have unilaterally decided to withhold his medications, they are interfering with the physician's recommended treatment and endangering his health. If the nurse cannot convince his parents to restart his prescribed medications, she should immediately report this to her nursing supervisor and the patient's physician.

In the past, families could rather easily have a family member committed involuntarily to a psychiatric facility. That began to change with the passage of the Community Mental Health Centers Act of 1963, which had as its goal the deinstitutionalization of psychiatric patients. This act, together with federal legislation establishing benefit programs that covered individuals with a mental disorder, and changes in laws that made involuntary hospitalization more difficult, led to the release of large numbers of hospitalized patients to live in the community. These social policies, conjoined with a growing emphasis on patients' rights, resulted in the establishment of the legal mandate to provide treatment that is the "least restrictive alternative." This requires that appropriate and effective treatment for mental illness be provided in the least restrictive setting. The restrictiveness of the treatment setting is evaluated in terms of the limits placed on physical freedom and the range of activities available to the patient. Halfway houses and total institutions like psychiatric hospitals impose greater restrictions that vary depending on the use of physical restraints, the amount of supervision, whether unsupervised private bathroom visits are permitted, and whether the patient is conferred adult status, which is signified by allowing a locked bedroom.

Because this patient can receive effective treatment for his illness in his parents' home, he has a moral and legal right to continue with treatment in that setting or a comparable one rather than the more restrictive setting of a psychiatric facility. If his parents are unwilling to cooperate in the prescribed treatment for his illness, the nurse should advocate for his placement in another setting that would constitute the least restrictive alternative. The nurse should not agree to help his parents have him committed to a psychiatric facility unless she believes that is necessary to protect his health.

The consequences for the family when a mental health patient lives at home should not be minimized. This family seems to be wrestling with two choices: give their son medications with perhaps unacceptable side effects or deal with the son's disruptive behavior when he does not take his medications. The harmful effects on the family may mean that treatment in a comparable setting should be considered, which the nurse could support.

Case 99

I have a patient who has a mental health problem that has not been controlled with medications. Recently he developed a serious medical problem and called me. I told him to call the paramedics; I was on the way. The problem was that he did not give me permission to share any information with the medical people. Can I say: "Don't transport him without restraints. He will try to jump out?" **How can I decide how much information I would be justified in sharing under these circumstances?**

The right to confidentiality of personal medical information is especially important for patients who have psychiatric diagnoses or substance abuse problems given the stigma that has historically attended these illnesses. Such highly confidential information can normally be disclosed to other health care providers only if the patient has signed a release granting permission to share information, or as required to protect his health and safety or to protect others. Confidentiality must always be overridden when it is necessary to protect the patient from serious, imminent harm. The decision about how much information to share should be governed by the condition that disclosure be limited to the minimum that is required in order to treat him effectively and safely. In the particular circumstances of this case, the nurse appears justified in informing the paramedics of the serious risks to her patient if he is not restrained, even without his permission.

Case 100

I have a bipolar patient who has been hospitalized multiple times for treatment because he is nonadherent with his medications. At times, he is the nastiest, most vicious person I ever met. He now has court-ordered, mandatory treatment, so I see him once a week to give him an injection. He always objects strenuously and tells me he doesn't want any injections. He also insists he doesn't want his family to know anything about his current problems. **What rights does he have if he is receiving mandatory treatment?**

Mental health patients may refuse medications or become nonadherent with a medication schedule because the side effects of many psychiatric drugs are difficult to tolerate. In fact, some patients stop taking medications as soon as their symptoms improve. Unfortunately, their illness can significantly worsen before they or others recognize that they need help. Nonadherence with medications is indeed the main cause of relapse and rehospitalization for patients with mental illnesses. Nurses thus have a particularly important obligation to teach patients about the need for psychiatric medications and to monitor their adherence to prescribed treatments.

Though this patient does not have the right to refuse his medication because his treatment has been court-ordered, he does have the rights of confidentiality and privacy. Both voluntary and involuntary patients retain the legal right to confidentiality of medical records, as well as the right to privileged communication. The latter is a subcategory of confidentiality referring to the statutory protection from disclosure of incriminating information revealed in the context of certain professional relationships. In *Jaffe* v. *Redmond*, the U.S. Supreme Court affirmed that a therapist need not disclose the content of therapy sessions even in a court of law. This protection has been extended in some states to the nurse-patient relationship.

Yet, there are exceptions to both privileged communication and confidentiality. The *Tarasoff* v. *Board of Regents* court decision found that health care professionals have a legal duty to warn of harm to specific others. The duty to warn has become the standard of care, following the requirements established by that decision.

THE PATIENT ADVOCACY ROLE

Case 101

My patient is a young woman who is a schizophrenic. She is also retarded. I want this woman to learn to read and to have some training so that she can work. I spoke to her mother about this, but her mother maintains that her daughter cannot work. She then confided she doesn't want her daughter to leave the house, and she doesn't want her to be near any men. She also told me she is concerned about losing the SSI check if her daughter works. I think her daughter would benefit from these programs. **What should I do when the caregiver's decision is not in the patient's best interest?**

When a patient such as this young woman does not have the capacity to make decisions, a family member normally is recognized as the surrogate decision maker, an arrangement that can be formalized through the appointment of the family member as a legal guardian for the patient. Surrogates should make decisions on the basis of substituted judgment when it is possible to know what the mental health patient values and what decision he or she would make if able to do so. Where that is not possible, as is the case with mentally retarded individuals who have never been competent, the standard of best interest must be used. A nurse must sometimes question the decision-making authority of a surrogate when a decision conflicts with the apparent best interest of the mental health patient. If it is necessary to take action to protect the patient, the nurse has the obligation to alert the appropriate authorities. A guardian or conservator should then be sought through legal proceedings.

As an advocate for this patient, the nurse should carefully assess the family caregiver's decision because it appears to oppose the patient's best interest. She should discuss this further with the patient's mother and provide information that addresses her concerns. Her mother may have underestimated the possibilities for her daughter, or she may have exaggerated the risks involved in participating in programs outside the home. If the mother continues to refuse to allow her daughter to receive training which would benefit her, however, the nurse should raise her concerns about the well-being of the patient with the daughter's physician and her supervisor.

Finally, the patient's mother has chosen to limit her daughter's social interactions and clearly intends to keep her at home, away from men. These decisions may violate her daughter's legal rights. Relevant here is the *Foy* v. *Greenblott* court decision, which established that every psychiatric patient has the right to individualized treatment under the least restrictive conditions feasible, posing minimized interference with a patient's individual autonomy and social interaction. As a consequence, mental health patients who are institutionalized have the right to privacy and personal association, which includes the right to have consensual sexual activity. Home health care patients presumably have the same rights.

Case 102

> The problem I have is with physicians who don't want their patients to see a psychiatrist. They tell a patient, "You don't need a psychiatrist. I'll prescribe something for your depression." They address the symptoms, but they don't try to solve the basic mental health problem. **What is my responsibility when this happens?**

Nurses have a responsibility to advocate for the services that they believe serve the best interest of the patient. This advocacy is particularly important for patients with mental health problems who are often subject to biased treatment and who may be unable to advocate effectively for themselves. When mental health patients would benefit from diagnosis and treatment by a specialist, the nurse's responsibility is to encourage the physician to make a referral to a psychiatrist or other specialist and to seek other mental health services as necessary, with the patient's consent. Unfortunately, getting patients access to care for mental health problems is particularly difficult under some insurance plans.

Case 103

I have a patient who keeps showing up at the emergency department with a complaint of shortness of breath and difficulty breathing. Her doctor is ignoring these complaints because she has a diagnosis of anxiety. I'm concerned that she may have chronic obstructive pulmonary disease. **What is my responsibility as a patient advocate?**

As an advocate for the patient, the American Nurses' Association Code of Ethics states, the nurse must take appropriate action if the rights or best interest of the patient are jeopardized by the practice of any member of the health care team. Accordingly, if the nurse believes that this physician is giving inadequate attention to the patient's symptoms, with possibly serious consequences, she has the responsibility to advocate on the patient's behalf. She should communicate her questions about the possibility of chronic obstructive pulmonary disease to the patient's physician and express her concern about the threat to the patient's health as clearly and as forcefully as she can. If that fails to produce the actions she believes necessary for her patient, she should report her concerns about inadequate care to her supervisor. The role of patient advocate is of special importance if physicians or other care-givers demonstrate a bias toward mental health patients, dismissing a patient's complaints, judging their symptoms to be less serious than obvious physical symptoms, or denying them access to services.

Nurses must be capable of effectively communicating the basis and urgency of various needs of a patient to other health care professionals and should document that specific assessments were provided to the physician. This is particularly important because nurses are legally responsible for informing physicians of their assessments.

SPECIAL RESPONSIBILITIES

Case 104

I have a Hispanic patient with posttraumatic stress syndrome. He has recently started seeing a cultural healer who dispenses herbal treatments; he said it's for the spirits. He doesn't think he needs any other treatments. I'm worried that he will take too much of these herbal treatments. Who knows what that will do to him? **Should I ask his physician to have treatment mandated to protect him?**

An acceptable response to this patient's decisions about treatment for his posttraumatic stress syndrome should begin with an assessment of the patient's cultural beliefs. Cultural competence is particularly important when caring for mental health patients because some cultures deny the very existence of mental illness, while others recognize mental illness but reject Western ideas about appropriate treatment. Indeed, mental illness is believed to have religious significance in some cultures. The phenomena of speaking in voices, trance-like conversion experiences, and the display of extreme emotion may be considered important expressions of religious fervor. The person who exhibits unusual thought patterns or behavior may be seen as chosen by God, someone who is to be honored and protected rather than subjected to medical treatment. There are other traditions which associate mental illness with negative forces, such as Satan, or see it as punishment for sin. Some place the blame for mental illness on the evil eye, a curse, or a hex. In such traditions, the mentally ill are often avoided or even banished from society. The treatments of Western medicine are believed to be ineffective and unnecessary responses to mental illness in many of these cultures.

Nurses should provide culturally competent care, which requires knowledge of the particular beliefs of a patient's cultural group, as well as the mental health symptoms that are commonly attributed to culturally-specific syndromes. Developing cultural competence will also help nurses understand the attitudes of families and community caregivers when patients suffer from mental illness. Although nurses should advocate for effective, safe treatment, they should also attempt to accommodate cultural beliefs concerning mental illness and should accept cultural practices that are not dangerous for the patient, provided that those practices do not interfere with any recommended treatments.

The patient in Case 104 undeniably has the right to make the decision to use herbal treatments instead of the prescribed Western treatment. The nurse's responsibility is to inform him of the risks of forgoing the recommended treatment and substituting herbal treatments, including the possibility that his condition will worsen significantly. Nevertheless, because there is no evidence that the patient is dangerous to himself or to others, there is no basis for asking the physician to seek court-ordered treatment. It would be an unjustifiable paternalistic intervention to seek treatment for the patient's own good in circumstances where the patient has the capacity to determine for himself what is in his interest.

Case 105

I'm concerned about my patients' safety all the time, and I mean all the time. I cross my fingers and hold my breath that the way I left them will be okay until I can get back for my next visit. One of my patients is on medication for anxiety, and I am there to monitor her medications and assess her mental health status. She has been suicidal. With suicidal patients, I am always afraid; I wonder if I can trust them and if they will tell me when they have thoughts of suicide. **How do I know the patient is telling me the truth if she says she is fine and doesn't think about suicide anymore? What is my responsibility in this case?**

When caring for mental health patients who may be suicidal, nurses have several specific responsibilities. The nurse's first responsibility is to assess the patient's mental health and the threat of suicide carefully and to seek hospitalization if necessary to protect the patient. Second, nurses have a legal duty to warn and must take action to protect others threatened with harm. Third, they must disclose a patient's intention to commit suicide or to harm others to other professionals involved in the care of the patient. Finally, nurses must document these concerns and any measures they have taken to reduce the danger.

Caring for suicidal patients presents several challenges. Critical to the successful assessment of mental health problems and the evaluation of the effectiveness of treatment when patients are suicidal is the ability to trust the information the patient provides. Further, the possibility that a patient would conceal thoughts of death or suicide, or deceive caregivers about how well they are doing, may complicate the establishment of a trusting nurse-patient relationship as a basis for providing nursing care. As a result of their mental health problems, moreover, these patients may not be motivated to follow recommended treatment plans or may stop taking the medications that have been prescribed for them, thus endangering their health. Consequently, with suicidal patients who are particularly vulnerable to harm, the professional obligation to act to protect patients' safety takes on added significance.

Where there is uncertainty about the patient's actual mental health status and a lack of trust in the patient's own assessments, the responsibility of determining whether it is necessary to seek hospitalization for the patient may be daunting. The nurse's responsibility in situations such as Case 105 is to assess the patient's mental health and alert the physician if there are reliable indications that the patient is not being truthful or that her condition is much worse than she admits.

Though these issues may arise with patients with terminal illnesses who are clinically depressed and perhaps suicidal, it is not as common for psychiatric nurses to be involved in the care of terminally ill patients at home. Dying patients are usually getting psychiatric home health care only if they are already being treated for mental health problems when a terminal illness develops, in which case one nurse usually provides both medical and mental health care. They may also receive mental health services if hospice becomes involved in their end-of-life care, since hospices have mental health professionals who are available as needed.

MANDATORY TREATMENT

Case 106

My patient has a horrible abuse history. Her father sexually and physically abused her. She had his baby when she was fifteen. He took the baby from her as soon as it was born, and she never saw the baby again. She has constant flashbacks, she is full of hatred and anger, and she repeatedly threatens to commit suicide. I don't think she will ever do it, but I'm not sure. That's what bothers me. **How certain should I be that a patient is dangerous to herself to justify a recommendation for mandatory treatment?**

A patient who is dangerous to herself can be subject to court-mandated treatment. This may include hospitalization, but it could mean that an individual receives treatment as an outpatient. Home health care nurses have the responsibility to assess whether the circumstances of a particular patient present such a risk and make a recommendation to a patient's physician.

With patients who may be suicidal, the difficulty is in judging whether suicide threats are credible and thus justify mandatory treatment. Though the nurse in this case has concluded that the patient's suicide threats are not credible, she is not certain of that assessment. It may appear then that she should recommend mandatory treatment for the patient's own good given her professional obligation to act to protect the patient. Yet, in the face of her uncertainty about the danger that exists, the decision to recommend mandatory treatment is morally problematic. The moral difficulty arises from the conflict between a competent patient's right of self-determination which assigns decisions about treatment to the patient herself, and the best interest of the patient which may require treatment against her will. Because the nurse also has an obligation to promote patient rights, she could attempt to persuade this patient to accept voluntary hospitalization or additional outpatient treatment for her mental health problems. This would respect the patient's right to make her own decisions about treatment while promoting her safety and health. If the patient refuses and the nurse remains uncertain about the danger, she should inform the woman's physician of these concerns and seek further evaluation of the patient. Mandatory treatment should only be sought when other options have been exhausted and the danger to the patient appears to be imminent and serious.

The moral difficulty of the situation would justify contacting the agency's ethics committee for advice and help in weighing the pros and cons of the alternative courses of action. As in all such cases, nurses should carefully document their concerns and any actions they have taken.

Case 107

My patient had previously been treated for an anxiety disorder that was diagnosed after she expressed suicidal thoughts. Two weeks ago she gave birth to a daughter. Her husband moved out soon after she came home from the hospital. I went to her home to do an assessment. Her house was completely dark. As I was interviewing her, she said, "I'm losing it." I expressed my concern that she was experiencing postpartum depression, but the patient said she is worried that if she agrees to treatment she will lose custody of her daughter. **Should I recommend mandatory treatment even though she will probably lose custody of her daughter?**

A recommendation for mandatory treatment would appear to be justified, given that there may be a serious risk of harm to the infant or to the patient. The nurse has a legal duty to warn of harm to another, following the requirements established by the *Tarasoff* court decision, in addition to the duty to warn of threatened suicide. Accordingly, the nurse has the obligation to notify child protective services about the possible danger to the baby and recommend immediate removal of the infant if her judgment is that the baby is in imminent danger. That will result in at least a temporary loss of custody, but the nurse really has no choice in this situation.

In the home health care setting, involuntary treatment often results when a patient is unable to recognize the seriousness of a mental health problem, for instance in cases of anorexia nervosa or court-ordered treatment following a Driving Under the Influence conviction. The patient may not believe that treatment is necessary and refuse to consent, with the consequence that treatment must then be mandated if there is risk to the patient or others.

Case 108

I have been caring for a patient with a history of depression who was just released from the hospital where she had been treated for congestive heart failure and cellulitis. She has bottles of pills everywhere in her apartment. Some bottles have only two or three pills; others are almost full. Old prescriptions for depression and expired medications for problems she no longer has are mixed in with her new prescriptions for her heart condition. There is no way to tell what she is actually taking. I did a mini-mental exam that convinced me she is severely cognitively impaired, though she insists that she can take care of herself. I don't think she will recognize that she's in trouble until it's too late. **Should a cognitively impaired patient have treatment mandated to protect her?**

Generally, treatment for mental health problems can be mandated for competent patients who are judged dangerous to self or to others and for patients who are incompetent, who can have treatment imposed if it is in their best interest. Some states also identify a category of patient known as "gravely disabled." Those who are classified as gravely disabled are unable to provide food, shelter, and clothing for themselves due to mental illness. The gravely disabled are deemed incompetent and therefore can be legally treated against their will.

Determining whether a patient has the capacity to make decisions is the crucial issue in many cases when assessing whether treatment should be mandated. To demonstrate their competence, adult patients must be capable of completing written forms outlining treatment and discharge plans (with help given to those with reading, sight, hearing, or speech impairment), and they must be able to repeat the treatment options, along with the benefits and burdens of each. A patient's capacity may be compromised if cognitive impairment precludes the ability to acquire new information or weigh the advantages and disadvantages of treatment options, including treatment refusal.

This patient's serious cognitive impairment may render her incompetent. That depends on whether she can in fact explain her medications and the dosages she should take. If she cannot do that, the nurse should take the appropriate steps to begin the process of having her incompetence demonstrated so that treatment in her best interest can be mandated. This requires a probable cause hearing to determine whether she should be treated against her will. In the interim, the nurse should help her to destroy any old and expired medications to diminish the risks. It is also important for the nurse to document her concerns and attempts to prevent harm to the patient to establish her efforts to meet her professional obligations.

Case 109

I have one dual diagnosis patient that I see weekly for court-ordered injections. Dual diagnosis patients are individuals who are diagnosed with a mental health problem who also have a diagnosis of substance abuse. These patients are really challenging. If you were dealing with a paranoid schizophrenic, you would know how to calm them down in a crisis situation. A paranoid schizophrenic with a cocaine habit is a different story because their perception is unique. You can't predict what they might do. That's the situation with this patient. He's unpredictable and he frightens me. **Would I be justified in leaving a patient's home if I am uncomfortable?**

Nurses accept an ethical commitment to care for patients without bias against any disease or particular health problem, implicitly acknowledging that they may be expected to provide care for people others stigmatize or to accept the risks of caring for individuals with infectious diseases, as an example. However, though nurses are expected to accept some unavoidable risks in providing care, they have the right to take reasonable actions in order to protect themselves. As is true when caring for other patients, nurses who take care of the mentally ill have the right to withdraw from a case provided that they adhere to agency policies. The nurse in Case 109 is certainly justified in leaving a situation that makes her uncomfortable as long as she makes the necessary arrangements to assure that the patient receives the care he requires. One possible solution is to return with a police escort to administer his injection. She should also document this situation and inform her supervisor of her concern that this patient may be dangerous.

ANALYSIS OF CASE 93

Case 93 involves a patient with dementia who is disturbing residents of his apartment house. The behavior of this elderly man affects the well-being of others, which raises an issue about the rights mental health patients have and the limits that can be imposed to protect the interests of other people.

Competent patients who have been diagnosed with mental health problems generally have the same rights as other patients. The diagnosis itself does not mean that they are incompetent. Accordingly, they have the right to make the decision whether to seek treatment, to accept or refuse medication, and to determine who has access to personal medical information. As is true for all competent individuals, they also have the right to make other significant decisions about their lives for themselves, including the decision about where they will live.

Nonetheless, competent patients can have mental health treatment mandated if they are deemed dangerous to self or others. In addition, some states classify patients as "gravely disabled" if they are unable to provide food, shelter, and clothing for themselves. Such patients are deemed incompetent and can be legally treated against their will. At this time, this patient does not appear to be gravely disabled, incompetent, dangerous to self or others. Moreover, he is entitled to receive mental health treatment that is effective in the least restrictive environment. For those reasons, he has the right to decide to continue living independently.

The nurse should monitor this situation as closely as she can so that she can continue to assess the patient's capacity to make decisions and respond if he loses capacity. She also must alert his physician if he appears to need hospitalization for treatment of his illness. Moreover, the consequences of the patient's dementia and hallucinations could become more serious. The other tenants of this apartment building have the right to insist on measures to protect them from any possible harm from this patient.

It should be noted that the nurse cannot reveal personal medical information about this patient to his landlord. That violates his moral right to confidentiality, as well as violating the requirements of the Health Insurance Portability and Accountability Act of 1996 and the specific regulations in most states governing the release of information about mental health patients.

ETHICAL CRITERIA

- A competent mental health patient has the right to make free, deliberate, and informed decisions, including the right to refuse treatment.
- The mental health patient has the right to truthful disclosure of information at an appropriate level.
- The mental health patient has the right to privacy and confidentiality of personal medical information.

PRACTICAL STRATEGIES

When a nurse is concerned about the mental health patient's vulnerability to harm:

- Take steps to minimize risks for the patient.
- Assess the need for intervention.

- Support the right of competent patients to make decisions.
- Monitor the situation for increasing dangers.

When others suggest withholding information from mental health patients:

- Advocate for truthful disclosure.
- Ensure that relevant material is presented to the patient in an understandable manner.

When a patient's family presents an obstacle to effective treatment:

- Educate the family about the best treatment for the patient.
- Remind the family of the patient's right to make treatment decisions.
- Encourage shared decision making.
- Report instances of suspected abuse.

When issues of whether to reveal confidential information arise:

- Protect confidentiality as far as possible.
- Disclose only what is necessary to protect the patient's health and safety or the safety of others.
- Review the legal requirements for nurses.

When patients suffering from mental health problems receive inadequate resources:

- Act to safeguard the patient.
- Advocate for expanded access to address the patient's needs.
- Report incompetent professional care.

When mental health patients are nonadherent:

- Attempt to determine the reasons for nonadherence.
- Reinforce the need for the treatment.
- Accommodate cultural beliefs and practices to the extent possible.
- Seek mandatory treatment if necessary.

When patients are suicidal or a danger to self or others:

- Encourage truthful disclosure.
- Evaluate the patient's need for hospitalization.
- Contact appropriate authorities in cases of psychiatric emergency.
- Act in accord with the duty to warn.
- Document steps taken to address safety issues.

Chapter 10

CARING FOR CHILDREN

Nurses share the care of children with parents, but parents are the primary decision-makers for their children. Ethical issues arise when a nurse questions a decision that seems to put at risk the health or well-being of the child.

Case 110

My patient is a three-year-old child who has been comatose for three weeks. She has a brain tumor that basically takes up the whole brain. Because she is on Dilantin, she is getting home health care. The family wants to continue aggressive care, but I think that aggressive care is only prolonging the girl's suffering. **Who should make these decisions for dying children?**

General Issues

- **Who should make decisions for children?**
- **What special responsibilities do nurses have when their patients are children?**
- **When may treatment be withheld or withdrawn from a dying child?**

INTRODUCTION

Though teams of nurses, physicians, and technicians provide the professional care children require when they are hospitalized, parents are expected to accept a substantial role when children are cared for

174

in the home. If children are developmentally disabled, chronically ill, or seriously injured, parents must learn to perform intricate tasks such as managing high-tech life-support systems. In addition, painful procedures that are performed by nurses and physicians in the hospital may be assigned to parents. They may be forced into the position of inflicting pain on their children by giving injections or suctioning a tracheotomy tube, for example. As a result, their role in home health care may be profoundly upsetting for parents. The relationship parents have with their children may be harmed as well, if children believe they can no longer trust their parents not to hurt them.

The dual roles of parent and caregiver consequently produce significant anxiety and distress. Adding to parents' distress is their sense that they have been forced to share control of their children's lives and well-being with outsiders who impose intrusive schedules and procedures. This stress is exacerbated when parents also have significant concerns about their other children and the ultimate prospects for the family in these circumstances.

Nurses strive to empower parents and families so that they have a sense of control and are able to cope with the tasks and burdens of caregiving. They attempt to establish a collaborative nurse-family relationship, which is the key to the successful care of children in this setting. Given the vulnerability of children, however, it may be quite difficult for home health care nurses to relinquish control of their care to parents or families if they appear to be ill suited to these tasks. Their uneasiness about the care families provide or the decisions they make for their children are the source of particularly troubling issues for nurses who care for children.

MAKING DECISIONS FOR CHILDREN

Case 111

I'm caring for a microcephalic girl who has a progressive orthopedic deformity. As she grows, her shoulders are moving forward and her body is curving inward. She is already having trouble breathing; she just had to have a bigger trach implanted. Eventually she will smother if nothing more is done. Her mother wants to put her on a ventilator when it becomes necessary. I don't agree with her about this. **What should I do when I disagree with parents about what is best for their child?**

Decisions about their children are the legitimate right of competent parents as long as the decisions do not constitute neglect or abuse. This child's mother has made the decision that, despite the ultimate outcome being unavoidable, she wants her child to be placed on a ventilator to assist her breathing, which will enable her to live longer. However, being dependent on a ventilator as breathing becomes increasingly difficult will involve suffering that could otherwise be prevented.

Nurses who disagree with the decisions parents make for their children can appropriately respond by providing information that is relevant to the decision. In this case, the nurse knows that the use of a ventilator will cause some suffering for this child, and it is appropriate for her to educate the parents about these consequences. As an advocate for the child patient, the nurse should promote what she believes to be in the child's best interest. In the final analysis, though, the mother has the right to make the decision to have her daughter placed on a ventilator.

The best interest of the patient standard is a deceptively simple-sounding principle, for well-meaning parties may have genuine disagreement about what constitutes the best interest. When this happens, the substantive issue about best interest gives way to the procedural issue of who is the lawful decision maker. Parents have the legal right to make these decisions, but if the parents are in disagreement with each other, it may be necessary to seek court intervention to determine what should be done.

Case 112

I have been caring for a young child who has been tested and found to be retarded. The doctor hasn't told the parents what the diagnosis is. Now the child's mother is asking me questions: "What do you think is wrong?" **Should I tell her what I know?**

In most cases, parents must give their permission, the equivalent of an adult's informed consent, for medical treatment of their children. Informed consent, in turn, requires having the information necessary to make an informed decision. Physicians must disclose children's diagnoses, treatment options, side effects, and expected outcomes to their parents.

Though full disclosure is necessary, this physician has not adequately disclosed the test results and the child's diagnosis. Lacking this information, the child's parents cannot make good decisions for their child. Moreover, they have been left with troubling uncertainty about their child's health when they deserve answers to their questions about what is wrong. To answer the mother's immediate question, the nurse can provide information about developmental stages, for example, and suggest sources of information that may respond to the mother's concerns. She should also encourage the parents to ask their questions directly of the physician, and she should advocate with the physician for a clearer and fuller explanation of the child's diagnosis.

Sometimes, despite the best efforts to inform them, parents seem to be in denial about the truth of their child's condition. Some parents believe that a miracle will happen and their child will be cured of his or her impairment. In such cases, there is not much that can be done other than to monitor the situation to be sure the child is receiving appropriate care.

Case 113

I have a case right now where the baby had meningitis and is vent dependent. The mother is a seventeen-year-old girl who insisted she wanted to bring the baby home to care for him herself. Her own mother called me to tell me that the girl doesn't take very good care of her baby. She had a doctor's appointment for the baby this week, but she made the decision that he didn't need to be seen. She skipped the appointment, so her mother wanted me to stop at the house to check on the baby. Then she said: "Don't tell my daughter I called." **Should this teenager be making decisions for this baby?**

Parents are recognized, morally and legally, as the natural decision makers for their children. They are assumed to know what is best for the child and to have the child's best interest at heart. Even in ordinary circumstances, though, this responsibility for making decisions for children can be overwhelming at first, especially if the parents are young and inexperienced. Further, when children are impaired or suffer from a chronic illness, the decisions required on their behalf become more complex and, subsequently, more daunting. Parents often lack the medical background to appreciate the full implications of the various options in cases like this. At the same time, they must cope with the emotional strain of adjusting to the reality that their baby is medically fragile. Some would argue that parents should not even be asked to make decisions under these circumstances.

A mother would be recognized as the natural decision maker for her baby; nonetheless, it seems inappropriate to place the full responsibility for difficult decisions on a parent who is a teenager. The nurse should instead encourage this young mother to seek the collaboration of others in making these decisions. The baby's grandmother, who has voiced her concerns about the baby, may be willing to share some responsibility for the care of this infant. Through shared decision making, the teenager and her mother could seek to make decisions that address the realities of the care required for an infant who is ventilator dependent.

Even if this teenager rejects the idea of involving her own mother, the nurse should continue to emphasize the advantages of shared decision making. She could suggest that this young mother seek someone else, for example, an aunt or a trusted older friend, with whom she could discuss her concerns and the decisions she must make. The nurse should answer any questions they have, clarify their options, and help them to identify the advantages and disadvantages of alternatives to assist them in the decision-making process. Ideally, this will ensure that good decisions will be made for the well-being of the infant, as well as sustain the relationship between the teenager and her infant son.

Also, the nurse could seek supplemental services. This mother will need help, because caring for a high-tech infant at home ordinarily requires at least two adults who are trained and available, in addition to the home health care nurse. However, if the grandmother's concerns about the care the infant is receiving are substantiated and demonstrate that there is a serious threat to the well-being of the infant, the nurse should report this to the appropriate authorities.

Case 114

I take care of an infant who has multiple neurological problems. The baby is extremely irritable. He cries when something touches him, he doesn't sleep, he can't stand to be held. In the beginning, even feeding the baby caused him to cry. The mother spends all her time trying to keep the baby content. They want to keep their baby at home, but the stress is evident. **Should I encourage them to try to find out-of-home placement for their child?**

Out-of-home placement usually appears to be a less desirable alternative for a child than remaining in the care of his family. The American Academy of Pediatrics has a policy which rests on the assumption that all children belong in families. One of the goals of the federal Healthy People 2010 Act is to reduce to zero the number of individuals with disabilities under the age of twenty-six who reside in congregate care.

Yet, recent surveys have shown that social services to help families cope are neither easy to access nor sufficient to meet the needs of many parents. Without willing, extended family nearby, continuing to care at home for a seriously impaired infant or child may present nearly impossible burdens.

Consequently, although home health care is often the best care for a child, it is not always feasible. In addition, home health care may not be substantially better care for this particular child, given his serious neurological impairments, if the child's level of awareness is so limited that he will not notice the loss of daily contact with his parents. Provided that is the case, the nurse could encourage the parents to seek alternative placement for their baby. She can lead the parents through a consideration of the burdens and benefits of out-of-home care versus home health care to help them reach a decision. This decision will most likely engender feelings of guilt and inadequacy in the parents, even if they believe it is a reasonable decision to make. The nurse can help them anticipate and deal with these negative feelings.

Case 115

I'm caring for a small child whose mother is a physical therapist. The physician ordered a medication for spasticity, with two units to be given, four times a day. The mother wants her son to have two and a half units, and she wants me to give it. She should understand that I can't do that, but she is insistent. **How should I deal with a parent who insists the medication dosage should be changed?**

As the primary decision makers for their children, parents are given considerable discretion. Parents are allowed to make decisions for their children that are less than the best decisions possible. They can even compromise the best interest of the child in order to accommodate what they see as the best interest of other members of the family. Moreover, when they must choose between treatment options, parents are allowed to choose or reject the recommendation of the health care team. Parents, for example, can refuse routine vaccinations for their children or use herbal remedies instead of other medicines to relieve cold symptoms.

However, the decisions that parents can make for their children are limited by law if the consequences are significant. For instance, though competent adults could decide to stop treatment for themselves, parents could not simply decide to stop life-saving medical treatment for their child. Legally, the standard of best interest of a child is said to be violated if a parental decision puts the child at risk of serious, imminent, and irreversible harm. In such cases, parental decisions may be overruled. This is true even in situations where the parents are acting in what they believe is the child's best interest. As an example, a Jehovah's Witness may want to refuse a life-saving blood transfusion for an injured child based on religious tenets. Nevertheless, the courts will override both the right to exercise religious freedom and parental authority to make medical decisions for one's children in order to meet the state's duty under *parens patriae* to protect innocent third parties and speak for those who cannot speak for themselves.

Parents with medical knowledge, as is the case here, may assume that they know best what medications and what dosages their child should receive. The nurse should question them to determine whether there are changes in the child's condition or a concern about side-effects or efficacy that is prompting the attempt to override the physician's order. This information could then be communicated to the physician so that he or she could decide whether to change the medications.

Unless there is a reason to question the physician's order, the nurse must administer the prescribed medication dosage; otherwise she could fail to meet the standard of care, and subsequently, could be legally vulnerable to charges of malpractice. She clearly cannot acquiesce to the mother's demands. When parents themselves alter a medication dosage or refuse to give it, the nurse must assess whether this is an example of medical neglect or abuse, which must be reported to the appropriate authorities.

Case 116

I am caring for a young girl whose mother has a significant anxiety disorder that prevents her from holding a job or going to school. She seems to be taking good care of her daughter, though sometimes her judgment is bizarre. Recently she has been insisting that her daughter wear heavy wool clothing even on the hottest days of summer. I'm concerned about her judgment, but if I report these concerns and she is hospitalized, she will probably lose custody of her daughter. She would be devastated by that and her own health would probably deteriorate. **When should we say that a parent is no longer capable of making decisions for a child? Should the child's interests take precedence over the interests of her mother?**

The safety and welfare of a child patient must always be the primary concern of nurses and others involved with the care of a child. If the competence of the parent or family caregiver comes into question, nurses have a clear responsibility to report the situation. Even though the consequence may be that the mother loses custody, decision-making and care must be turned over to someone else if there is real risk to the child.

Nurses should exercise their responsibility to assess an individual's mental health and a possible need for hospitalization with great care, nonetheless. In this case the consequences of recommending hospitalization would be far-reaching and serious for both the child and her mother. To diminish the risks and the need for hospitalization, the nurse could attempt to discuss her concerns with the mother and suggest she contact her own physician for an evaluation of her health. She should continue to monitor the situation so that she can take more aggressive steps if the mother's judgment and behavior deteriorates.

There are a number of other ways in which safety concerns arise in pediatric home health care. Sometimes the home itself is unsafe for anyone. In other cases, the child has particular needs that cannot be met in the home, for example, when a child with respiratory problems lives in a house where temperature, animal dander, and dust cannot be properly controlled. Other family members can pose safety risks to an ill child if they smoke.

In response to these concerns about the safety of children, nurses should intensify their efforts to educate the family about the risks, contact the physician if necessary, and report to child protective services when appropriate. State agencies may sometimes seem slow to respond or reluctant to take action. Nonetheless, nurses must perse-vere in these efforts if their professional assessment is that the child is unsafe in the home.

SPECIAL RESPONSIBILITIES TO CHILD PATIENTS

Case 117

I have a patient with brain cancer who is a teenager. Though his parents know he's dying, they won't let us address this with the patient. They won't even let the chaplain come in to see him. He's been asking me questions, but one of the parents is always in the room and they step in and stop the discussion. I think he'd like honest answers, but they won't allow it. **Should children be told the truth?**

Since minors are not allowed to make any medical decisions, it may seem that they do not need to be told the truth. After all, the legal basis for requiring truthful disclosure is to promote an informed decision, and, generally, minors do not have the legal right to give informed consent to medical treatment. Except in special circumstances, parents or guardians must give proxy consent for minors. Because parents are presumed to act in the best interest of their children, courts endow them with broad decision-making authority. The government or courts can restrict parents' rights only if they have a compelling inter-est, such as the preservation of life and the prevention of suicide, safe-guarding against physical or emotional abuse or neglect, the protec-tion of innocent third parties, or maintaining the integrity of the med-ical profession. Otherwise, parents have the right to raise their chil-dren as they see fit.

There are several circumstances, however, in which minors are allowed to consent for themselves. For purely pragmatic reasons, most states allow minors to give their own consent for conditions that pose risks to public health and which might go untreated if the minor had to get parental consent. These include treatment for substance abuse and venereal disease. Some minors have the legal status of emanci-pated minors, meaning that they have all the rights and responsibili-ties of adults. This status is conferred if they are in the armed forces, or married, or if they have proven they have economic independence from their parents. In addition, some states recognize certain individuals as mature minors for the purpose of consenting to their own treatment. This usually follows the recommendation of a physician who testifies that they can demonstrate an understanding of the nature and consequences of treatment or refusal and can exercise the judgment of an adult.

A less formal substitute for informed consent is the requirement of informed assent. Federal regulations require that children over the age of seven be informed about their treatment in age-appropriate language and be asked for their assent. Even without assent, beneficial treatment can be provided for children if parents provide their consent. Only in nontherapeutic research does a child's refusal to assent serve as a veto to the child's participation in the research.

Despite the fact that minors cannot ordinarily consent to medical treatment, it does not seem right to withhold the truth from them, especially when older children who possess the decision-making capabilities of an adult ask questions about their health. Nurses may also believe, in other particular instances, that their minor patients should be more fully informed about their health and the medical treatments they are receiving. Some people maintain that even young children have the right to know about their illnesses in language suited to their age. Parents, though, have the right to decide how much information, if any, is disclosed to their children. Even when parents have decided to withhold all information from a minor patient, nurses should not lie or deceive a child, though they are expected to refrain from volunteering information to a young child. They should defer to parents to answer any significant questions children have.

A compelling case can be made for truthfulness when the patient is a teenager, as in Case 117. Given the fact that he is persistently questioning the nurse and seems to want honest answers, the nurse should advocate for disclosure of information. She may also want to discuss with the parents the advantages of promoting his understanding so that he can openly discuss his concerns and fears, and contribute to the end-of-life decisions that will be required on his behalf. Nonetheless, the decision to disclose information is the parents' decision to make.

Case 118

When teenagers become pregnant, nurses are sometimes dealing with issues such as sexually transmitted diseases and promiscuity. Another nurse told me about a teenager who was pregnant, reportedly by the same boy who is the father of my patient's baby. I wanted to say: "She should be treated for chlamydia" because I know the other girls he got pregnant. **What exactly would I be justified in revealing in this situation?**

Medical information must be kept confidential, even information about babies, children, and teenagers. This is required because all patients have the moral and legal right of confidentiality, a right which is recognized in the HIPAA regulations governing privacy of personal medical information. Accordingly, information about the paternity of a patient's child or about her health normally should not be shared with others, even other nurses, unless they are involved in her care. Confidentiality of such information can justifiably be breached only on the grounds that it is required by law or necessary to prevent harm. Granted that revealing the risk of chlamydia to another nurse might be justified for that reason, the issue is how much should be revealed to other health care professionals and, further, whether that information should be shared with the teenager's parents.

Because parents are the legitimate decision makers for their children, most feel they have the right to know everything about them. However, for purely pragmatic reasons, most states now grant minors over a certain age the right to confidential medical care concerning family planning, treatment of sexually transmitted diseases, and substance abuse. Otherwise, without the promise of confidentiality, minors are likely to go untreated, with disastrous consequences for themselves and public health. The parents of the pregnant teenager therefore should not be informed that she may be at risk of chlamydia. Moreover, the nurse does not need to reveal the risk of chlamydia to the other nurse because pregnant adolescents are routinely screened for sexually transmitted diseases. There is thus no justification for revealing any information at all about her own patient to another nurse who is not involved in this patient's care.

Parents and minors have the right to expect that information about the health of all family members will be kept confidential. The only exceptions would be the same as those for adults. Certain communicable diseases that pose a public health threat must be reported, along with suspicions of child abuse and any injuries that suggest criminal battery, such as gunshot and stab wounds. Generally, information can only be released to schools, insurance companies, or others concerned with the care of the child with the parents' consent.

Case 119

I have a case where the parents are completely overwhelmed. Their son was born with multiple physical and cognitive handicaps, and now that he's getting bigger, he's more difficult to care for. The stress is having a significant effect on the family. I'm beginning to suspect that the husband is hitting his wife. I observed two ugly bruises on her arm the last time I was there, but she denied that there was any violence. This last week they forgot to give their son his medications twice. My concern is that their child is not getting the care he needs under these circumstances. **What is my responsibility in this case?**

Nurses have special responsibilities when their patient is a child who cannot advocate for himself. When parents are not carrying out the plan of care, this may be reportable as child neglect. There are two questions that can help a nurse to determine whether or not to report parents as neglectful: (1) Is the child at real risk? Are the parents making decisions that are genuinely harmful to the child? and (2) Would the child be better off staying with this family or being placed somewhere else? Given the difficulty of finding good placement for children with special needs, these questions should be considered carefully. The response of child protective agencies is often frustrating because investigations are sometimes cursory and agencies may appear to do nothing to address the concerns about child neglect. Moreover, such agencies are reluctant to separate children and parents, especially when alternative care for the child with special needs is difficult to arrange.

When families fail to comply with the plan of care, it is essential to inquire about their reasons for neglecting the medications and procedures that have been prescribed. Nonadherence may be the unintentional result of an increasingly stressful situation when parents carry the emotional and physical burden of caring for a seriously ill or handicapped child. Nurses can assist parents in finding the resources available to them to help them cope with the burdens of providing this care. Respite care is available in many communities, as an example, to help parents in exactly these kinds of circumstances.

Unfortunately, one of the greatest problems parents face is learning about and gaining access to services. State, federal, and private practical help may be available, but complex bureaucracies and inadequate information about these programs are sometimes insurmountable obstacles for families to negotiate. For example, the Katie Beckett Waiver allows Medicaid funding for the home health care of children, regardless of parents' income or resources, if the child's disability is so severe as to require "institutional level care." But parents often need assistance in applying to this kind of program. Nurses are an excellent resource for parents because they can provide information and link families to the right agencies or connect them with a social worker who can help them.

It is well documented that the divorce rate of parents of children with chronic illness or psychological or developmental problems is much higher than average. Child abuse or domestic violence may also be a result of the frustration, stress, and disruption of the home that such families encounter. If evidence of child abuse or domestic violence exists, nurses should report this to the appropriate authorities.

Case 120

> My patient is a four-year-old child who nearly drowned. She is very, very fragile. She is NPO, that is, she is not to have anything by mouth. The problem is that her parents want her to have the same experiences other children have, so they have been feeding her anyway. I tried to explain to them that this is dangerous for her, but they think it is important that she be able to eat food like other children can. **Should I do anything else?**

Parents understandably want to provide their handicapped children with the typical experiences of childhood, as far as that is possible. Indeed, many of these efforts are beneficial to the child and the family, but some are not. Though being able to feed their child has important symbolic meaning for parents, this is very risky for the child, for feeding a ventilator-dependent toddler by mouth poses a real danger of aspiration. The nurse should again attempt to convince the parents of the dangers involved, and she must report this to the child's physician. No nurse will condone or cooperate with such medically dangerous behavior. In her absence, unfortunately, the child is vulnerable to whatever the parents do in the privacy of their home.

Case 121

I am working with a family that is totally noncompliant, which is affecting my eight-year-old patient's health. This child is incontinent of stool and urine when she is angry, so she has to wear pull-ups. I'm there to give enemas and monitor her diet. She lives with her grandmother who has given up. She is not monitoring the girl's medication; instead, she expects the child to do that herself. There is no money for the special high fiber diet the physician recommended, so she is not on the right diet. This girl needs a structured routine, which she is not getting either. **How can I care for a child whose family refuses to cooperate?**

Children with serious health problems are particularly vulnerable if they are being raised by family members with limited emotional and financial resources. Their families may be unable to consistently meet their responsibilities as caregivers or to supply what the child needs in order to be healthy. Additionally, motivating a child to stay on the medication prescribed for behavioral problems, which can be very effective, is frequently a challenge. Without the cooperation of their families, children often fail to get the proper medication. Families may also fail to provide the emotional support that enhances a child's health.

Unfortunately, community resources for caring for children who have serious medical and behavioral problems are stretched thin. Child psychiatrists are in short supply in many communities, with the result that there are long waiting periods before a child can be seen and assessed. Consequently, many children who would benefit from psychiatric evaluation and treatment, or whose health would improve if they were temporarily living in a structured environment, such as a facility with a staff of trained child care workers and therapists, do not get the help they need.

In this case, intervention is clearly needed. State agencies should be contacted and a plea made for better arrangements for this child. Unless there is evident neglect or abuse, however, state authorities may be limited in the actions they can take to improve the child's situation.

Case 122

I am involved in caring for a two-month-old boy who is an anencephalic. Everything that is possible has been done to keep him alive this long. His parents, who are Muslims, believe he needs to be circumcised to go to heaven. His doctors refuse to do the procedure because they are concerned that he might hemorrhage and die. The boy's parents are angry and extremely upset. **How can I be a successful advocate for this family?**

Even when their children are receiving home health care, the parents of infants with serious impairments often seem to be at the mercy of the medical system. They may believe the system prevents them from caring for their children as they see fit, especially when physicians refuse to perform a procedure or prescribe a medication a parent wants. On the other hand, parents should not be able to "order" medical treatment; nurses and doctors are not mere technicians assigned to carry out whatever procedures patients or parents want. This means that the parents do not have the right to demand that the physicians carry out the circumcision. The physicians can reasonably refuse, on the basis of their professional judgment that it poses an unacceptable risk of harm for this baby.

Granted that this infant will not survive long even with the best of care, the claim that circumcision poses an unacceptable risk is debatable. But the disagreement between parents and physicians goes deeper than that, for this case presents a real clash of values. The view that physical survival is most important clashes with the belief that the life of the spirit is more valuable. The tradition of Western medicine clearly favors physical well-being and makes little accommodation for parents with different values.

To advocate for this baby and his parents, the nurse could suggest finding a different physician who would be more willing to carry out the parents' wishes. She could also suggest that the parents consult their religious leaders to determine whether an exception to the requirement is possible in the specific circumstances of their infant. Some religions, for example, exempt hemophiliacs from being circumcised. Many religious leaders in the United States have found ways to accommodate their religious practices to the requirements of Western medicine. Discussing this with their religious leaders may result in a solution to the clash of values between parents and physicians.

Case 123

Some families believe that everything that happens is God's will and don't believe in major medical interventions. One of my cases involves a baby who is very underweight for his age. He was born with a neurological impairment associated with some retardation, and he doesn't suck very well, so his nutrition is less than adequate. The doctors have suggested either a nasogastric tube or surgery to place a G-tube. Because his family has refused to give permission, the doctors think they should try to have the baby removed from the home so they can treat him. **Should I support the parents or the doctors in this case?**

From the perspective of this country's legal system, parents, physicians, and nurses are guilty of medical neglect if treatments are refused that could sustain or substantially improve the life of the child. Thus, if nontreatment poses a risk of substantial irreversible harm, parents can be required to accept it or lose custody of their child. Regardless of their own religious beliefs, parents must agree to the life-saving interventions Western medicine affords for their children.

There are some few exceptions where courts have allowed minority groups to be exempted from laws about children. In general, though, the state has an interest in children and stands *in loco parentis*, in the place of parents, to assure their welfare. The state will not hesitate to intervene on behalf of the child in life-threatening situations. Therefore, even though the parents are opposed on religious grounds, the nurse should support the physicians and the decision to perform surgery. She can try to help the parents understand that this surgery is legally required and attempt to help the family cope with the emotional burden of having medical procedures imposed on their child.

END-OF-LIFE DECISIONS

Case 124

I am caring for an infant who was born with very severe abnormalities. They basically sent him home from the hospital to die, but his parents can't "let go." They are waiting for a miracle. They insist that all his nurses agree to attempt to resuscitate him and call for emergency services if he arrests while they are there. **What is my responsibility? Should I agree to keep resuscitating him?**

For everyone involved, the decision to stop resuscitating an infant is wrenching. There is no clear-cut criterion outlining when it is ethically appropriate to withhold or withdraw a life-saving treatment from a very young child. Generally accepted policy for newborns considers these things: treatment may be withdrawn if the infant is chronically and irreversibly comatose, treatment would merely prolong dying, treatment would not be effective in correcting all of the life-threatening conditions, treatment would be futile in terms of physical survival, or treatment would be virtually futile and inhumane. Considerations of the infant's quality of life, such as whether the infant is capable of any kind of meaningful relationship or whether the balance of painful sensations far outweighs any pleasures, may also be cited as justification for these decisions. All of these criteria are controversial and open to interpretation.

If this infant is conscious and capable of suffering, withholding resuscitation and invasive treatment can be justified as a way to avoid pointless suffering. Also, his severe abnormalities could possibly justify such a decision on the basis of the infant's poor quality of life. Ultimately, continuing treatment of the infant under these circumstances amounts to using the child as a means to the parents' gratification and should not be encouraged.

However, the ethical situation is complicated. Parents have the right to decide that they wish to continue aggressive treatment, but physicians and nurses have no obligation to give futile or unnecessary treatment. Therefore, from a moral perspective, the nurse is not required to keep resuscitating this infant because resuscitation is futile. Agency policy, however, may dictate that nurses abide by the parents' wishes in such circumstances, but should allow the nurse to request to be taken off the case, if she is in serious disagreement with the parents' decisions.

Nurses can help families of dying children by explaining the role of palliative care specialists and pediatric hospice care. The transition from thinking in terms of cure to thinking in terms of care is often resisted by parents because they see it as "giving up" on their child. Explaining that giving up aggressive treatment is not abandoning the child but instead treating him in a different way, with the goal of relieving his pain and suffering, should help parents accept the situation. Sometimes parents are more accepting if organ donation is a possibility and they can see it as a way of validating the importance of their child's life.

Case 125

The patient is a five-year-old child with muscular dystrophy. Though he is deteriorating, his parents don't believe it. They want everything done for him. The nurses are in disagreement about this case. Some of his nurses are trying to convince the parents that we can't stop treatment now. I think they don't understand the dying process. I think we should let him go in peace. **Should I go along with all this aggressive treatment?**

Decisions about stopping treatment for children with terminal illnesses may be even more difficult for parents than deciding for newborns because the emotional attachment to the child is greater. Usually in such cases, decisions are based on an analysis of the burdens of treatment in terms of suffering and lowered quality of life, measured against the benefits of longer survival and enhanced quality of life. Nurses can advise, relying on past experience, but ultimately parents have to make the decision.

In some situations, a hospital-based nurse who has been caring for a critically ill child may "follow him home" and accept a position as a home health care nurse for the child. Parents might ask a nurse to become involved in this way, particularly when the nurse has cared for the child for several weeks in intensive care. When this happens, there could be disagreements between the nurses from the "hospital culture" who are used to focusing on cure and aggressive treatment and other home health care nurses. These differences should be discussed and resolved outside of the home setting and without involving the parents. This is also a situation where a nurse could consult with her agency supervisor to determine how to handle this kind of conflict. The agency's ethics committee would also be a useful forum for discussing issues of professional disagreement.

Case 126

It is so tough when a child is dying and he knows what is going on. I have a fifteen-year-old patient who has relapsed after a lot of chemotherapy. They have run out of options, and he is going downhill pretty fast. His parents let him make all the decisions, such as whether to try a new experimental drug, whether to go back to the hospital, or remain at home. I admire their trust in him, but I think they may be giving him too much responsibility. **Should I say something to them about it?**

Adolescents like this fifteen-year-old are not legally adults but they can often participate in life and death decisions. Whether he should be given complete responsibility is not as clear. The nurse can recommend that this family utilize shared decision making to reach these decisions. The patient would still have a significant role, but he would benefit from the insights and advice of his parents, and he would be able to share the responsibility for the tough choices. She should also talk to the patient to determine if he has any questions or concerns that she can answer and to help him clarify the values and preferences he has about his treatment.

Though the psychology of the dying child is complex, research shows that even quite young children may know and understand more about their condition and prognosis than adults realize. Children often have what is referred to as "closed awareness"- they know they are seriously ill, but they do not discuss it openly. Some families prefer to cope with serious illness and impending death in this way.

In other cases, children may want to discuss illness and death. Children who have chronic diseases frequently develop an understanding of their condition and a maturity that belies their chronological age. They may ask explicitly, "Am I going to die?" When caring for seriously ill children, nurses should discuss responses to this question with parents, and they should be prepared to respond tactfully but truthfully to children's questions. They can attempt to assure the child that he or she will not be abandoned and will not suffer. Finally, when children endure a long-term illness like cancer, at some point they may signify that they are tired of fighting the disease. The child's viewpoint should be taken seriously. Helping parents to listen to their children and to respect the perspective of a dying child is an important ethical role for nurses.

ANALYSIS OF CASE 110

Case 110 involves a three-year-old child with a brain tumor that has grown to take up virtually the whole brain. The nurse caring for this child disagrees with the parents' decision to continue aggressive treatment. Two separate issues about decisions for dying children emerge in this situation. The first is the question of who has the legitimate authority to make these decisions. The answer is clear because the right to make decisions for children is well established in practice and in law. Parents, whether biological or adoptive, are the designated decision-makers for their children. The legitimacy of the decision-making authority of competent parents becomes an issue only when there is evidence of abuse or neglect, or if life-saving medical treatment is refused for a child. In that event, the state will intervene to protect the child. When parents are not competent or if they have lost custody, they cannot make decisions for their children. A legal guardian can be appointed by a court. As an alternative, often grandparents or other family members are informally recognized as individuals who have the authority to make medical decisions for children when the parents are not able to do so.

The second issue in this case is to determine what decisions are justified when children are dying. That issue is best answered by looking at the consequences of the available choices for treatment. Most often, a calculation of the benefits and burdens will lead to a reasonable decision for a child with a terminal illness. There can, of course, be disagreement about consequences, because an analysis of benefits and burdens involves making predictions about the future. It is also true that people weigh the value of end results differently. Despite these complications, an evaluation of consequences is an appropriate method of ethical reasoning when someone must choose between alternative treatments for a dying child.

The nurse can assist the parents in reaching decisions that reflect the important values they have by offering to help them consider the consequences of pursuing aggressive treatment versus withdrawing treatment for their child. The burdens of aggressive treatment, such as the pain and suffering that may be experienced by the child, can be weighed against the benefits of a prolonged life, and compared to the burdens and benefits of withdrawing treatment. How these consequences are evaluated will depend on the parents' basic values. Helping the parents to analyze the benefits and burdens of alternative treatments may provide a way for the nurse to understand their decisions for their child and may reconcile her to the choice they have made. In the final analysis, though, the nurse must defer to whatever decisions the parents make unless their decisions raise issues about neglect or abuse. These decisions are difficult personal matters, and it is the parents who should have the ultimate authority to determine the end-of-life care for their child.

ETHICAL CRITERIA

- Children over the age of seven have the right to be informed about their treatment in age-appropriate language and to give assent to the treatment.
- Parents have the right to make decisions about medical treatment for their minor children and are entitled to request beneficial treatment even without a child's assent.
- Parents have the right to withhold or withdraw life-sustaining treatment from their children under certain circumstances.

PRACTICAL STRATEGIES

When the nurse disagrees with the family about what is in the child's best interest:

- Advocate for the child.
- Educate parents about the consequences of their choices.
- Contact the physician and agency supervisor.
- Raise ethical concerns with the agency's ethics committee.
- Seek court intervention, if necessary.

When physicians withhold information from parents:

- Encourage parents to ask questions directly of physicians.
- Advocate with the physician for a clearer and fuller explanation of a child's diagnosis.
- Avoid deception.
- Provide educational materials that respond to parents' concerns.

When concerns arise regarding the ability of parents to make decisions for their children:

- Assess the risk and act to safeguard the child.
- Support the parents' efforts to act in the best interest of their children.
- Educate the parents about available resources.

- Contact the agency supervisor.
- Report medical abuse and neglect to the authorities.

When providing home health care becomes overwhelming for parents:

- Advocate for access to care that best meets the needs of the patient.
- Facilitate decision making regarding burdens and benefits of out-of-home care.
- Recommend counseling services to support the family.
- Contact the agency's social worker to advise parents about community support services.

When parents' cultural and religious values dictate nonstandard care for their children:

- Assess whether there is a threat of serious harm.
- Ensure that the parents understand the medical consequences and legal implications of their decisions.
- Suggest a consultation with religious leaders, if relevant.
- Report cases of abuse and neglect to the proper authorities.

When parents request futile or aggressive treatment for a dying child:

- Explain the conditions under which it is legally permissible to withhold or withdraw life-sustaining treatment.
- Support the parents' emotional needs and explain the role of palliative care.
- Enlist the help of a social worker and identify community resources.
- Consult the agency's ethics committee.

APPENDICES

Appendix A

LEGAL RULINGS

Contents

Arato v. *Avedon*
Supreme Court of California, En Banc, 1993
S. Cal. 4th 1172, 23 Cal. Rptr. 2d 131, 858 P. 2d 589

The case against Dr. Avedon brought by Miklos Arato's family raises questions concerning the exact nature of informed consent, when information is material to a patient, the limits of therapeutic privilege, and whether it is ever morally and legally wrong for a physician to give a patient too much hope.

The widow and children of Miklos Arato, who died of pancreatic cancer, brought action against his treating physicians, claiming that they breached their duty to obtain informed consent for treatment by failing to disclose information regarding the life expectancy of pancreatic cancer patients. Miklos Arato was a successful electrical contractor and real estate developer when he was diagnosed with pancreatic cancer at the age of forty-two. Under the advice of his physicians, Arato undertook aggressive treatment for his cancer, including radical surgery, chemotherapy, and radiation.

Testimony indicated that Arato was informed by his physicians that pancreatic cancer is usually fatal, told about the unproven nature of the proposed treatment, and in light of that, the option of foregoing treatment altogether. Before his initial meeting with the team of oncologists, Arato had filled out a questionnaire with one hundred and fifty questions. Among them was a question about whether patients wanted to be told the truth or whether they wanted the physician to bear the burden for them. In spite of the fact that Arato made clear that he wanted to be told the truth about his condition, his physicians did not disclose to him the statistical life expectancy data for patients with pancreatic cancer.

The physicians claimed this information was not material. Material information consists of information that physicians know or should know would be regarded as significant by a reasonable person in the patient's position when deciding to accept or reject a recommended medical procedure. Such information is needed to make informed decisions regarding proposed treatment. The patient's family claimed that had Arato known about the statistical morbidity associated with his disease, he would not have wasted his time undergoing treatment but instead would have spent his remaining months enjoying his family and arranging his business affairs. The false hope that led him to agree to treatment was a result of negligence on the part of the physicians, according to the Arato family.

Mr. Arato's treating physicians justified not disclosing statistical life expectancy data to their patient for various reasons. His surgeon testified that Mr. Arato had experienced a great deal of anxiety over his condition, to the extent that the surgeon was convinced that it would have been medically inappropriate to disclose specific mortality rates. Arato's chief oncologist, Dr. Melvin Avedon, contended along different lines that cancer patients "wanted to be told the truth, but did not want a cold shower." He argued that the direct and specific disclosure of extremely high mortality could deprive a patient of any hope of cure, which was medically inadvisable. Further, the physicians pointed to what little value predictive statistics were when applied to a particular patient with individualized symptoms, medical history, character traits, and other variables. They also testified that neither Mr. Arato nor his wife ever asked for information concerning his life expectancy in more than seventy visits over a period of a year.

The Supreme Court held that (1) physicians did not have a duty as a matter of law to disclose statistical life expectancy data; (2) evidence supported jury's finding that physicians reasonably disclosed information material to patient's decision; (3) physicians did not have duty to disclose information material to patient's nonmedical interests; (4) expert testimony regarding disclosure of statistical life expectancy data was admissible; and (5) erroneous jury instruction on physicians' duty was not reversible error. The court also held that the propriety of disclosing life expectancy information to a cancer patient depends on the standard of practice within the medical community.

In the Matter of Karen Quinlan, an Alleged Incompetent
Supreme Court of New Jersey, 70 N.J. 10, 355A 2d 647

The case of Karen Ann Quinlan was instrumental in establishing the right to refuse life-sustaining treatment under privacy rights against unwanted bodily intrusion. Since Karen was in a persistent vegetative state, this case was also significant in establishing the rights of guardians to discontinue extraordinary treatment used to prolong the life of an incompetent patient, without charges of homicide or wrongful death resulting.

On April 13, 1975, twenty-one-year-old Karen Ann Quinlan had been celebrating with friends at a birthday party when, after a few drinks, she began to pass out. Thinking Karen was drunk, her friends helped her into bed so that she could "sleep it off." However, later that evening, when they went to check on her, Karen was found unconscious and no longer breathing. Two of her friends attempted mouth-to-mouth resuscitation and then rushed her to the hospital early in the morning on April 14th. Though she was found to have drugs and alcohol in her system, the levels were insufficient to have caused either a toxic or fatal reaction. Although the cause remained undetermined, Karen nevertheless had somehow suffered brain damage from oxygen deprivation, rendering her irreversibly comatose.

Karen's parents and sister and brother initially held out hope for a recovery. Karen seemed responsive to light and sounds at times. She would open and close her eyes, grimace, and make chewing motions. In spite of this, her condition rapidly deteriorated. Karen, who was five feet and two inches, dropped from one hundred and twenty pounds to seventy pounds and contracted into a fetal position. Her breathing was being done with the assistance of a respirator that had been placed in her throat after the doctors had performed a tracheotomy.

Karen's physicians at St. Claire's Hospital, Dr. Robert Morse and Dr. Arshad Javed, were in agreement that there was no reasonable hope of recovery from her coma. Further, even if she did make some physiological improvement, the overall quality of her life would remain the same. Three-and-a-half months after Karen was hospitalized, the family was reconciled to the fact that she would never regain consciousness. They also knew that she would not want to be kept alive under the circumstances. Yet, before making a decision to request discontinuing treatment, Joseph Quinlan, Karen's father, visited his parish priest. The priest, Father Thomas Trapasso, explained the Catholic Church's position that there is no moral duty to use extraordinary means to keep a person alive. Now convinced that it was God's will that Karen be allowed to die, Joseph Quinlan went to the physicians and granted permission to have her removed from life support. On July 31st, the Quinlans provided written authorization to discontinue Karen's treatment and agreed not to hold the hospital liable for the outcome.

Although Dr. Morse assured the Quinlans that they were doing the right thing, the next morning he contacted them saying that he had changed his mind and could no longer go along with the removal of the respirator. One explanation for Dr. Morse's dramatic change of heart came from the hospital attorney who had notified the physicians that because Karen was legally an adult, Joseph and Julia Quinlan were no longer her legal guardians. In order for them to make the decision to refuse treatment on her behalf, they would need to seek legal guardianship in a court of law. Karen's father, therefore, went to court in an effort to be appointed guardian of the person and property of his daughter. If granted, guardianship would authorize him to discontinue all extraordinary medical procedures purportedly sustaining Karen's life. These measures, he asserted, presented no hope of her eventual recovery. In addition, there was no financial incentive for the family to request removal of treatment since Medicare was paying the $450 a day to keep Karen alive.

Quinlan's attorney, Paul Armstrong, appealed to three constitutional principles: (1) the right to privacy, (2) religious freedom, and (3) cruel and unusual punishment. The right to privacy, Armstrong claimed, includes the right against unwanted bodily intrusion. This allows patients and their guardians to refuse even life-sustaining treatment. The question to be addressed was whether the state's interests in the preservation of life and the prevention of suicide were compelling enough in this case to override the liberty and privacy interests against unwanted bodily intrusion.

Because Joseph Quinlan believed he was acting in accordance with the doctrines of his Catholic religion, Armstrong also argued on the grounds of religious freedom. To deny Quinlan the opportunity to act in accordance with these principles by having life support for Karen discontinued would violate Quinlan's First Amendment right to religious freedom.

Finally, Armstrong argued that to keep Karen alive under the circumstances would violate her human dignity and constitute a form of cruel and unusual punishment in violation of the Eighth Amendment.

Judge Robert Muir of the New Jersey Superior Court ruled against Joseph Quinlan's petition on November 10, 1975. Muir found the state's interest in the preservation of human life overriding. Even though she was in a persistent vegetative state with no chance of ever regaining consciousness, because Karen had measurable brain activity, she could not be declared legally dead under the Harvard Brain Death Criteria. Because of that, Judge Muir considered the removal of treatment intended to end her life as an act of homicide and euthanasia. Though he did not question the good faith and motives of Mr.

Quinlan, he believed Quinlan was too emotionally involved and distraught over Karen's condition to be appointed guardian.

Quinlan's attorney appealed Judge Muir's ruling to the New Jersey Supreme Court. Chief Justice Hughes described the significance of the case as follows:

> The matter is of transcendent importance, involving questions related to the definition and existence of death, the prolongation of life through artificial means developed by medical technology undreamed of in past generations of the practice of the healing arts; the impact of such durationally indeterminate and artificial life prolongation on the rights of the incompetent, her family and society in general; the bearing of constitutional right and the scope of judicial responsibility, as to the appropriate response of an equity court of justice to the extraordinary prayer for relief of the plaintiff.

Hughes ruled in favor of Mr. Quinlan, allowing him to assert a privacy right on behalf of his daughter. At the same time, he set aside any criminal liability that might result from removal of Karen from the respirator. He also suggested that the family consult with the St. Claire's Ethics Committee to determine whether there was agreement with the prognosis. Following a meeting with the Ethics Committee, Karen's physicians at St. Claire's weaned her off of the respirator. They did, however, express their intention to put her back on if there were signs of respiratory distress. They made clear that they did not want Karen to die under their care from the removal of the respirator, as they expected would happen. For this reason, the Quinlans had Karen moved to the Morris View Nursing Home. She remained there until her death on June 11, 1985.

Superintendent of Belchertown State School v. *Saikewicz* 370 N.E. 2d 417 (Mass. Supreme Court 1977)

The case of Joseph Saikewicz was instrumental in extending the right to refuse treatment to both competent and incompetent patients under certain circumstances.

Joseph Saikewicz was sixty-seven-years old and severely retarded, with an I.Q. of ten and a mental age of two years and eight months, when he was diagnosed with acute myeloblastic leukemia. He had been institutionalized for the past fifty-three years and had been a resident of the Belchertown State School since 1928. Apart from the leukemia, Saikewicz was physically strong and in good general health. His severe retardation rendered him incapable of verbal communication, however, leading him to resort to grunts and gestures to express himself. One result was that Saikewicz was unable to respond to even simple questions regarding his medical condition, such as inquiries about whether he was experiencing pain. The only living relatives who could be located were two sisters who declined involvement in his case. Therefore, the superintendent of the school went to court requesting a guardian *ad litem* be appointed to make decisions on behalf of Saikewicz to determine whether he should undergo a course of chemotherapy. Given his age, stature, ability to participate in treatment and the stage of his illness, it was estimated that the treatment offered a 30 to 50 percent chance of remission, with a return of the disease in two to thirteen months. The disease will ultimately be fatal.

The guardian *ad litem* and Saikewicz's two attending physicians recommended against chemotherapy on the grounds that the burdens of treatment would outweigh the benefits. Although most patients with this diagnosis opt for chemotherapy, they accept the burdens with an understanding of the possible benefits. The hope, therefore, provides some measure of comfort. In the case of Saikewicz, he would experience the fear and physical discomfort of chemotherapy without being cognizant of the fact that it might be useful in prolonging his life. Moreover, the extension of his life was both uncertain and limited. Under the circumstances, Saikewicz's guardian was convinced that imposing treatment would be cruel.

There were three fundamental matters addressed by the Court in this case: (1) the nature of the right of any person, competent or incompetent, to refuse potentially life-sustaining treatment; (2) the legal standards that must be used to determine whether life-sustaining, though not life-saving, treatment should be administered to an incompetent individual; and (3) the procedures that are necessary to follow in arriving at the decision.

The Court ruled that the right to refuse life-sustaining treatment extends to both competent and incompetent individuals. The judge viewed the decision by the guardian to refuse treatment as consistent with the prevailing position in medical ethics that treatment should not be imposed when it offers no hope of recovery, where recovery refers not only to the ability to remain alive, but also to a life without intolerable suffering. He weighed the interests of Saikewicz in refusing treatment against the state's interests in: (1) the preservation of life; (2) the protection of the interests of innocent third parties; (3) the prevention of suicide; and (4) maintaining the ethical integrity of the medical profession. The judge allowed Saikewicz's guardian to refuse treatment on his behalf under an appeal to the "best interests" principle.

Cruzan v. *Director, Missouri Dept. of Health* 110 S. Ct. 2841, 1990.

In 1990, the U.S. Supreme Court for the first time made explicit reference to "a right to die" in its discussion of the now familiar case of Nancy Cruzan. In a 5–4 ruling, the Supreme Court recognized a strong constitutional basis for living wills and the designation of another person to act as a surrogate for medical decision making. The ruling was based on an appeal to liberty interests outlined in the Fourteenth Amendment to the Constitution. The Constitution also permits states, according to Judge Rehnquist in the majority opinion, to decide on the standard that must be met in determining the wishes of comatose patients.

Nancy Cruzan was twenty-four-years old when she lost control of her car around midnight on an isolated, icy country road in Missouri on January 11, 1983. She was thrown thirty-five feet from the car and landed facedown in a water-filled ditch. A farmer noticed the headlights shining across his field and alerted the authorities. By the time paramedics were able to reach her, Cruzan's heart had stopped. The paramedics were able to restart her heart, but because she had been without oxygen for approximately fifteen minutes, Cruzan remained in a persistent vegetative state. For the next seven years, there was no change in Cruzan's condition. Because she was unable to swallow, she remained alive only with the help of feeding and hydration tubes. Unlike the case of Karen Ann Quinlan, however, which had become famous a decade and a half earlier, Cruzan did not need a ventilator. Thus, removal of the feeding tubes became the central issue in the Cruzan case.

In 1988, Judge Charles Teel of the Jasper County Circuit Court heard testimony from Nancy's parents, Louise and Joe Cruzan, and her sister, Christy, that Nancy said on many occasions she would not want to live under these circumstances. Judge Teel ruled in favor of their petition and granted the right to remove the feeding and hydration tubes based on the right to liberty of individuals to refuse death-prolonging treatment.

However, the Missouri Supreme Court in a 4–3 decision overrode the lower court's ruling. The reason was the state's living will statute that specifically forbade the withholding of food and water to hasten death. Judge Teel had argued in the lower court that Cruzan nevertheless retained the right to remove the surgically implanted tube used to administer food and water. But, because the Cruzans had not provided clear and convincing evidence that Nancy would have found the tube burdensome and intolerable, the judges found the state's interest in the preservation of life compelling in this case.

On June 25, 1990, the Supreme Court ruled that competent individuals retain a significant liberty interest in remaining free from unwanted bodily intrusion. In this case, the use of technology led to a sustaining of life that actually interfered with individual liberty. Addressing the issue of incompetent patients, the Court set a standard for clear and convincing evidence regarding patients' wishes concerning treatment refusal under the circumstances. Therefore, the Supreme Court refused to reject the legal standard set by the state of Missouri, which would have overturned the appellate court's decision. Nevertheless, they left the door open for the Cruzans to go back to the Circuit Court and provide the clear and convincing evidence required to demonstrate that Nancy would have found the feeding tubes intolerable. On December 14, 1990, Judge Teel accepted the evidence offered by family and friends of Nancy Cruzan and ordered the feeding and hydration tubes removed. Cruzan died twelve days after the removal of the tubes on December 26, 1990.

In the same year that the Supreme Court made a decision in the Cruzan case, federal legislation was passed aimed at protecting the rights of patients in such medical crises. The Patient Self-Determination Act of 1990 mandates that each patient be informed of the right to exercise treatment preferences, including preferences concerning life-sustaining measures.

The Case of Joyce Brown v. *Mayor Ed Koch*
Court of Appeals of New York, 10 N.Y. 2d972

This case illustrates some of the challenges associated with assessing dangerousness and outlines the various conditions that must be met under governmental powers to involuntarily commit those who suffer from mental illness.

Joyce Brown, known to the public as "Billie Boggs," became famous for being at the center of a legal battle to determine the rights of the mentally ill against involuntary commitment. Boggs was a forty-year-old who survived on the streets of New York City. To the dismay of those she encountered in the affluent Manhattan neighborhood whose streets she wandered, Boggs engaged in a range of bizarre behaviors, some of which were violent. She would expose herself, speak in rhymes that were sexual in content, and tear up money and urinate on it. She was often filthy and smelled of urine and excrement. Mayor Koch's administration had implemented a program known as "Project Help" to evaluate homeless mentally ill individuals for potential psychiatric treatment. Boggs's actions and lifestyle prompted the concern of emergency psychiatric services personnel, who diagnosed her as suffering from serious mental illness. Social service employees at New York City Health and Hospital Corporation sought to have Boggs involuntarily committed for treatment. This action was vehemently opposed by the New York Civil Liberties Union, which argued that Boggs was in her current plight due to homelessness rather than significant mental illness. The Civil Liberties Union contended that forced evaluation leading to involuntary commitment would surely violate the rights of the mentally ill. On October 28, 1987, Boggs was forcibly removed from the street and brought to the emergency room at Bellevue Hospital. She was treated and moved to a locked psychiatric ward. She called the ACLU from there, and their lawyers agreed to represent her on the condition that they could use her story to publicize the plight of the homeless.

When Boggs's story was broadcast on television, three women came forward and identified her as their sister. They told the story of a bright, happy, attractive child from New Jersey who was a successful student and business school graduate. She worked for both Bell Laboratories and the New Jersey Human Rights Commission before becoming dependent on heroin and cocaine. During this same time, she was diagnosed as psychotic and involuntarily committed by her sisters for treatment. When she was released two weeks later, she went to the east side of Manhattan and began living on the streets.

Traditionally, two governmental powers have been applied to justify involuntarily treatment of individuals with significant mental illness. The first is the police power that is invoked by governments to protect citizens from the harmful actions of others. The second is the power of *parens patriae.* The state is parent to its citizens and as such is responsible for the care of those who are unable to care for themselves, including the mentally disabled.

In meeting its duties toward citizens, the state uses both criminal and civil commitment to promote safety and welfare. Further, civil commitment of an individual who suffers from mental illness has been justified by appeal to both powers to protect the individual from harming herself and to prevent harm from coming to others. Thus, there were two sections of New York's Mental Hygiene Law that could have been applied. Under the *parens patriae* statute, the state needed to demonstrate that Boggs suffered from a mental illness and that treatment in a hospital was appropriate, her welfare was impaired, and she was incapable of understanding her need for treatment.

However, in Boggs's case, a more stringent standard was agreed upon by the court. Beyond meeting the conditions necessary under *parens patriae,* the state required the H.H.C. to demonstrate the likelihood of serious harm to self or others. The proof of dangerousness was necessary to invoke the use of police powers to achieve civil commitment.

Conflicting testimony of experts provided little guidance for the judge, Robert Lippman, who ultimately relied on his own assessment of Boggs and ordered her released. A five-judge appeals court found Lippman in error (3–2) and accepted H.H.C.'s proof of dangerousness. Yet, because Boggs was entitled to refuse psychotropic medication, she was released from the hospital on the grounds that without treatment, it would serve no purpose.

Boggs became a celebrity for a while, accepting job offers and television appearances, and speaking at law schools on behalf of the homeless. She ended up back on the streets, however, all the while maintaining that she was not insane, simply homeless.

Warthen v. Toms River Community Memorial Hospital
101 N.J. 255, 501 A.2d 926 N.J., 1985

A nurse's primary responsibility as a patient advocate will, at times, lead to conflicts between a nurse's ethical duty to her patients and the legal duty she has to her employer and the physician. Such conflicts pose the potential for serious professional risk. A nurse who is ordered by a physician to perform acts she considers unethical or which are illegal or not in the best interest of the patient must decide personally and professionally how much to risk for the sake of practicing nursing according to the standards she has set for herself. Conflicting rulings in the courts provide little guidance for nurses in assessing these risks. Nevertheless, there are cases that provide an outline of how the courts have dealt with employer's efforts to limit the nurse's role as a patient advocate.

One of the mostly highly publicized cases was *Warthen* v. *Toms River Community Memorial Hospital.* Corrine Warthen worked as a nurse specialist in kidney dialysis at Toms River Community Memorial Hospital in New Jersey. She was assigned to dialyze a terminally ill double-amputee patient who was in renal failure. On two prior occasions, Warthen was forced to halt the procedure because the patient suffered both severe internal hemorrhaging and cardiac arrest. Warthen was opposed to further dialysis for this patient on moral grounds. In accordance with the ANA Code, she notified her supervisor in a timely manner of her objections to performing a procedure that she opposed morally and professionally. Warthen was convinced that further treatment was not in the patient's best interest. She attempted to appeal to the ANA code to justify her refusal of care on the grounds that the code mandates respect for human dignity. Warthen believed the patient's human dignity was violated by continued attempts at dialysis. When Warthen was fired, she used a public policy defense to make a claim of wrongful discharge.

According to the employment-at-will doctrine, employment can be terminated by either party without there being a cause for legal action. Warthen was seeking an exception to this doctrine on the grounds that when she failed to follow orders, she was acting justifiably in accordance with her professional code. There was legal precedent for such an appeal. In *Pierce* v. *Ortho Pharmaceutical Corp.*, the court recognized that professional employees owe a special duty to abide by the recognized codes of ethics within their professions, as well as to state and federal laws. However, the court held that an employee has a cause for action for wrongful discharge only when the discharge is contrary to a "clear mandate" of public policy. The burden of proof is on the employee to identify the expression of public policy in the code. The court found against Warthen because her acts, although done for the sake of the patient, could not be shown to benefit the public to such an extent that they would constitute a public policy exception to the employment-at-will doctrine. Public policy exceptions are based on the premise that allowing the employer to fire the employee under the circumstances would go against the public good and should therefore be prohibited. New Jersey's Supreme Court had also just passed a law upholding patients' rights to expect that medical treatment will not be terminated against their will. The court was concerned about potential conflicts if nurses were allowed to withdraw from cases for moral reasons. Patients' rights, the court insisted, must remain paramount.

The implications of this case for the home health care nurse are far-reaching. Like Warthen, a nurse may be acting from conscience out of concern for patient welfare and safety. Further, because of the importance of the nurse-patient relationship, a nurse's role as advocate may legitimately fall under the purview of public welfare. Yet, this is not sufficient to provide the clear mandate sought by the courts. In the absence of state statutes and case law supporting nurses' acts of refusal, the nurse is left without legal protection from dismissal by the agency and perhaps even loss of her license.

Lampe v. *Presbyterian Medical Center*
41 Colo. App. 465 P 2d. 513, 1978

In the case of Lampe v. Presbyterian Medical Center, the plaintiff, who was the head nurse of an intensive care unit, brought suit against her employer for retaliatory discharge on the grounds that her termination violated a mandate of the Colorado Nurse Practice Act. This case sheds light on the status of professional codes for nurses in courts of law.

The plaintiff, Lampe, was responsible for staffing the intensive care unit at the Presbyterian Medical Center. When she was ordered to reduce overtime expenditures, she refused to do so out of fear of jeopardizing the health and safety of her patients. Lampe was subsequently fired for her unwillingness "to fulfill the requirements of her job description."

Lampe appealed to her state's Nurse Practice Acts, which required a nurse to act in a manner consistent with the health and safety of her patients. According to Lampe, if she had followed orders to reduce the overtime of her staff, she would have violated the statute under which she was licensed. However, the court refused to recognize the Nurse Practice Acts as sufficient to "modify the contractual relationships between hospitals and their employees in such situations."

The dilemma faced by Lampe is a familiar one for home health care nurses who practice in a time of managed care. Home health care nurses are often torn between an agency's mandate to visit a certain number of patients within a short period of time and the needs of patients who require lengthier, more frequent, or continued visits.

Tuma v. Board of Nursing
100 Idaho 74, 593 P. 2d 711, 1979

The Nurse Practice Acts have been used by both sides in claims of wrongful discharge by nurses acting in their roles as patient advocates. This case centers on the limits of that role and the issue of whether providing a patient with requested information about alternative treatments for cancer constitutes unprofessional conduct in violation of the Nurse Practice Acts.

In *Tuma* v. *Board of Nursing*, Tuma, a clinical nursing instructor, requested the assignment of administering chemotherapy to a patient with leukemia. Tuma was concerned about addressing the needs of dying patients. This particular patient reportedly pleaded with Tuma to return in the evening, after the treatment, to discuss an alternative to the chemotherapy. Tuma agreed and discussed the possibility of laetrile and dietary therapy with the patient. Unfortunately, the patient died two weeks later as a result of experiencing serious adverse side effects from the chemotherapy.

Although no one contended at the trial that Tuma's actions in any way caused harm to the patient, hospital personnel contacted the Idaho State Board of Nursing and complained that Tuma had interfered with the physician-patient relationship. A hearing officer concluded that Tuma's discussion of treatment alternatives with her patient did in fact constitute unprofessional conduct in violation of the Idaho Nurse Practice Act. The Board of Nursing upheld the hearing officer's decision and suspended Tuma's license for six months.

Tuma won her case on appeal. The Idaho Supreme Court cited the Minimum Standards, Rules, and Regulations put forth by the Idaho Board of Nursing, which require nurses to promote patient education based on the individual's health needs. Tuma's actions were consistent with this mandate. Therefore, the court held that the Board of Nursing violated Tuma's rights by authorizing the suspension of her license in the absence of a specific statutory definition of what constitutes unprofessional conduct.

Home health care nurses, in their role as patient advocate, should be familiar with the laws in their state covering nursing practice and the extent and limitations of the protections provided by state statute and other public policy mandates. The Nurse Practice Acts are often too vague and broad to provide clear guidance to the courts. As a consequence, nurses who believe they are doing what is required of them as a nurse can be subject to disciplinary action, including dismissal, without any recourse in the courts.

Tarasoff v. *Board of Regents of University of California* 529 P. 2d 553 CA, 1976.

Tarasoff v. *Board of Regents of University of California has had a substantial impact in relation to the law surrounding misfeasance—the duty to prevent harm. The resulting ruling from this case was that the duty to confidentiality must be breached when there is a threat of serious imminent harm to an innocent third party. While psychiatrists at the time of the decision were concerned about its effects on the willingness of patients to disclose information necessary for their treatment, their fears have proved unwarranted in the years following this case.*

Prosenjit Poddar became obsessed with nineteen-year-old Tatiana Tarasoff. After she made clear to Poddar that she had no interest in a relationship with him, he sought psychiatric care from a staff psychologist at the University of California's student counseling center. Poddar confessed homicidal thoughts to the psychologist, who immediately contacted campus security. The psychotherapist expressed concern regarding Poddar's dangerousness and requested involuntary commitment of Poddar for observation and treatment. Upon questioning by the police, Poddar promised to stay away from Tarasoff and convinced them that he posed no real danger to her or himself. He then discontinued counseling and, two months later, killed Tarasoff. Her parents successfully sued the University for both failure to detain Poddar and failure to warn their daughter. The court thus upheld a duty on the part of psychiatrists to warn innocent third parties of threats directed at them by psychiatric patients.

In re Baby K. 16 F. 3d. 590; 1994 U.S. Court of Appeals

The case of Baby K. raises important questions regarding what constitutes futile treatment and who should be allowed to make the determination. Baby K.

was born with anencephaly. The life expectancy for infants born with just a brain stem ranges from a few hours to a few weeks. Death usually results from respiratory failure due to the inability of the brain stem to regulate breathing. In spite of the fact that even if she were to survive, her daughter would never have the capacity for thought, Baby K.'s mother sought aggressive treatment against the wishes of health care providers.

Baby K., an anencephalic infant, was born in Fairfax Hospital in Falls Church, Virginia, in 1993. Her mother was told that the standard treatment for babies suffering from anencephaly is to be kept comfortable until their organ systems fail, which most often occurs within a few weeks. Baby K.'s mother, who had deeply held Christian beliefs that all life should be protected, wanted everything medically possible done for her child.

Baby K. was cared for in a nursing home. At sixteen months, she required two hospitalizations for respiratory problems. Following her second hospitalization, Fairfax Hospital went to court seeking a ruling that would allow them to refuse what the doctors considered to be futile treatment for Baby K., given that her medical condition would not improve as a result. In spite of a hospital ethics committee ruling in support of discontinuation of aggressive treatment, the district court found in favor of Baby K.'s mother.

The hospital, along with Baby K.'s father, appealed to the U.S. Court of Appeals. This court applied the standards of the Federal Emergency Medical Treatment Act, which prohibits the abandonment of individuals in medical emergencies. Even though Baby K.'s treatment exceeded the prevailing standards of medical care, the court ruled that there were no exceptions passed by Congress that would preclude treatment just because it might not be expected to provide a medical benefit. Thus, Baby K.'s mother won the right to have her treated against the wishes of physicians who considered the treatment futile.

Appendix B

ADDITIONAL CASES

Good ethical decisions require critical thinking at each step of the process, as the ethical issue is framed, possible solutions are identified, and reasons are evaluated. Judgment in weighing the relevant moral factors and skill in critical ethical thinking is developed through practice in applying ethical theory to specific cases. Additional cases are offered in this section.

Guidelines for Analysis and Discussion

1. Formulate the ethical issue as a question (there may be more than one issue in some cases.)

   Consider: Which features of the particular situation are significant? If there is not enough information provided, what questions should be asked?

2. Critically assess the moral factors that apply to the situation.

   Consider: What rights do the individuals involved have?
   Which relationships and responsibilities are significant?
   What are the likely consequences?
   What do moral ideals require?
   Finally, which moral factors should be given the most weight?

3. Propose answers to the ethical question and identify the reasons that support each answer.

4. Develop a consensus on what the nurse should do.

If there is disagreement or moral uncertainty, consider which reasons are more compelling to attempt to resolve the issue. Some disagreements may reflect basic differences in important values, with the result that there will be no consensus about what it would be right to do. In such cases, individuals may have to agree to disagree.

Cases

1. A hospice patient of mine has a pacemaker that will keep his heart beating and prolong the dying process. Would it be ethical to shut it off? What should I say if the patient asks my advice?

2. Sometimes patients on powerful pain medications present special problems. It is necessary to restrict the number of pills left in the house at any one time. When a patient dies, the family must dispose of the medications. The nurses are not supposed to do that unless the medications are in a pump. I had a case where I didn't realize the patient's son was a recovering addict since that was not in the medical record. He took his mother's death very hard. While I was in the other room making calls after she died, he swallowed half of each medication, liquid morphine and liquid Attavan. I had to call 911. Ideally, how should I have handled the situation? Should I have been told he was a recovering addict?

3. I was assigned to care for another nurse's patient when she went on vacation. He is an elderly man who has lived on his own for several years and has done well. More and more frequently now, however, he is forgetting to take his heart medication. I am seriously concerned about his safety, his living conditions, and his ability to keep up with his medication. I told the other nurse that someone should intervene to protect him. She said that he had been brought up in a rural area where people are used to being fiercely independent and that is important to him. She argued that he has the right to live as he wants. Which argument is more compelling?

4. I have a patient who is an amputee, a young veteran. His wife has no interest in doing anything for him and she lets him know that. He tries to cook for himself, but he doesn't eat right, and he doesn't take his insulin when he should, so he has had frequent hospitalizations. What are the limits of my professional obligation to care for this patient?

5. I had a patient with cancer of the tongue who required tube feedings from 8 p.m. to 8 a.m. The instructions said "15 drips a minute." His wife, in her eighties, was told "You really have to watch this. It's important." So she stayed up all night long watching it drip. What is my responsibility to the patient's wife?

6. I've been visiting a nice elderly Chinese-American woman who is recuperating from a bad fall. I have noticed clear signs of early Alzheimer's disease and advised her son that she should be checked for that. There are medications now and adult day care programs that she could benefit from. "Oh, no," he said, "we don't want anyone outside the family to know about this. My mother wouldn't want it." Should I respect their beliefs and leave it at that or should I pursue this with the son or the physician?

7. I am experiencing some conflicts about a young child who is on home ventilator therapy. Their doctor keeps encouraging the parents, saying that they are doing a good job of caring for him, but she doesn't see the toll it is taking on the family. The mother has given up her job, so there are money problems, and she worries constantly that something will go wrong. The other two children have had to take on responsibilities way beyond their years. Even if home care is the best situation for the child, shouldn't these other factors be taken into consideration? Will I be failing my responsibilities as an advocate for this child if I suggest moving him out of the home?

8. I have a young woman with sarcoma of the pelvis. She had surgery ten years ago and has been unable to walk for three years. She has a pump for the pain, but it is not enough. She is still in chronic pain. Her orthopedic doctor is very cold. When she complained, he threw a tissue at her and walked out. He won't return her calls or mine. I faxed him a form with the information about her chronic pain. He

just signed it and faxed it back, but he took no action. When I confronted him, he said, "Well, at least you have it documented that you did something." He won't let anyone else in his office take her case. Have I done all I should do for this woman?

9. We have been working with a woman for a year to get her to the point where she is willing to disclose her HIV status to her partner. She is afraid of his reaction because domestic violence is a big issue in their relationship. The physician and I plan to go to her home to talk to her and her partner. She wants us to say she just found out that she is HIV positive. Should we agree?

10. Just as I was leaving my patient's house yesterday, his granddaughter walked out with me and quietly began asking for advice about contraception. I didn't want to turn her away. She is almost eighteen and trying to be responsible, but she is not my patient. What should I have said?

Appendix C

ETHICS COMMITTEES IN HOME
HEALTH CARE AGENCIES

Introduction

A home health care agency should establish policies, procedures, and resources that promote ethical behavior and facilitate the resolution of ethical problems. Ethics committees are useful for advice and also provide important support for nurses when they contend with moral uncertainty or moral disagreement.

What Is an Ethics Committee?

An ethics committee is an advisory or consultative group which provides a forum for the discussion of ethical issues as they arise in clinical practice. It serves as a resource to clarify complex issues and help resolve incipient problems. In most cases, an ethics committee does not itself make decisions, which are the responsibility of patients, families, or professional staff.

Ethics committees began to develop in hospitals in the 1970s, following the Quinlan decision in which the court directed hospitals to establish committees to address situations which generate ethical questions. Currently, accrediting organizations such as the Joint Commission on Accreditation of Healthcare Organizations require institutions providing health care, including hospitals, hospices, and home health care agencies, to establish a process for consideration of ethical concerns. This requirement may be met by establishing an ethics committee.

What Do Ethics Committees Do?

Ethics committees typically have three functions. First, an ethics committee can provide a review of a case with the goal of resolving ethical issues. These issues may arise as a puzzle when a new or unusual situation arises and the nurse genuinely does not know what she ought to do. Alternatively, an issue may stem from a conflict between staff members or between staff and patients or families where there is a difference of opinion about the right thing to do.

Second, an ethics committee provides education about ethical policies, values, and principles for healthcare professionals. This education should promote ethical sensitivity, recognition of ethical issues, and sound reasoning about ethical issues. Healthcare professionals should develop the skills to become better able to resolve moral uncertainty and avoid ethical conflicts before they escalate.

Third, ethics committees can review agency policies, upon request, to ensure that these policies reflect patients' rights and nurses' rights. For example, there should be clear guidelines specifying when an agency can dismiss a patient from service or a nurse can withdraw from a particular case. These guidelines must be consistently applied and fair to everyone involved.

What Are the Advantages of Ethics Committees?

As technology evolves and new rules are established by third-party payers, novel ethical questions arise. Using an ethics committee as a forum for discussion should lead to a fuller understanding and consensus among staff about how to respond.

All agency employees who participate in ongoing ethics education sponsored by an ethics committee will develop skills in communicating with patients, families, physicians, and other nurses. Having a chance to articulate their own views and listen to the views of others prepares nurses for explaining, reasoning, and advocating when the actual situation arises. Participating in ethics education will also promote the recognition of the differences in values that may persist among individuals, even with good communication and extended discussion of an ethical issue. The values of others must be acknowledged and respected, an attitude that is developed through skillful ethics education. Finally, ethics education will help those participating to learn the important distinction between clinical questions and questions about values. In its educational function, the committee should reach out to all employees of the agency. Nurses, as well as certified nursing assistants, home health care aides, and others, if feasible, should all attend.

Ethics committees can contribute to the knowledge of all agency staff about ethical issues. They also will serve as an important resource on ethics for the healthcare organization when questions about policies and procedures or clinical cases arise.

Discussion of ethical issues, when carried out in a supportive and cooperative way, should improve collegiality, introduce new employees to the culture of the individual agency, and perhaps help prevent moral distress and burnout from what can be a stressful and fast-paced profession.

How to Set Up an Ethics Committee

Ideally, a home health care agency will establish relevant policies, a membership statement, and ethics committee procedures, which can be included in a manual made available to committee members. Small home health care agencies may decide to develop less formal policies and procedures but still should communicate with staff and patients the relevant ethics policies, the procedures governing the ethics committee process, and the appropriate uses of the ethics committee. These materials are recommended:

1. A **Policy** establishing the ethics committee that sets out the purpose of the committee and identifies the functions of the committee, which typically comprise education, advice on policies and policy development, and advice on clinical ethical issues. The policy should outline the procedure for accessing the committee for advice.

2. A **Membership Statement**, which should be part of the policy establishing the committee. Determine the areas that require representation, for example, hospice care, mental health, and maternal/child care. The committee should include at least one individual who specializes in ethics who does not need to be a religious leader. Perhaps new committees should include someone with ethics committee experience, for example, on a hospital ethics committee.

The membership statement should list the areas to be represented on the committee, the length of terms of service (staggered terms recommended), and the number of times the committee meets each year (quarterly meetings are suggested, with the possibility of additional meetings if required).

Agencies should be careful to establish an environment that encourages free discussion of ethical issues and viewpoints. A chairperson who has the trust of the staff and credibility with them is important so that the committee will be taken seriously. The chairperson of the committee need not and perhaps should not be the person with the highest rank, since ethics discussion should be an open process with various viewpoints represented. It should be clear that this is different from a process in which decisions are handed down by authorities. Most important, the staff must feel free to bring questions to the committee for discussion without fear of intimidation or reprisal.

Committee members should be protected under the agency's umbrella policy against malpractice, provided that appropriate actions are taken in accord with agency policy and procedures and the requirements of law and federal and state regulations.

3. **Procedures** which identify the required steps for requesting a meeting/consult with the committee. A brief form, to be completed in writing, could ask for the reason for the consult, the patient/case involved, and the person requesting the consult. The procedures should also identify the contact person for the committee who will receive the completed form and set the process in motion.

The committee may wish to conduct a "mock" consultation to educate committee members about the appropriate referrals and the procedures to follow. Consults are appropriate when there is moral uncertainty or disagreement about what is right to do. Ethics committees are not intended to serve as the "ethics police." Examples of ethical wrongdoing should be reported as required by law, regulations, or agency policies.

The procedures should set out the steps in the process of consultation with the committee and identify the results of consultation. The committee could offer an advisory opinion, recommend a meeting with representatives of the committee, or arrange a family/team meeting facilitated by committee members to discuss the issues.

4. A **Manual** should be provided to each member which includes the committee policies and procedures. The manual should also include relevant law, regulations and agency policies, such as HIPAA regulations and material on advance directives.

5. **Evaluation Procedures**. The committee should provide for an annual discussion of committee functions and membership, and review agency and committee policies and procedures. An annual educational program which addresses ethical issues of interest for home health care nurses and agency employees, as well as new policies and regulations, is recommended

6. **Suggested Policies for Home Health Care Agencies:**
   • Ethics Committee Policy
   • Confidentiality of Medical Information [HIPAA and agency procedures]
   • Advance Directives
   • End-of-Life Decision-Making, which would specify agency procedures for withdrawing care and address end-of-life decisions
   • Conflict Resolution Procedures
   • Whistleblowing Policy

Getting Started

One important ethics committee function is the review of cases which present ethical issues. A review of an actual clinical case drawn from the experiences of agency nurses would provide an excellent example for introducing committee members to the distinctions and values utilized in analysis and discussion of ethical issues. A resource person in the community could be enlisted to chair this first meeting, thus providing a role model of how such a committee works. Since all hospitals are required to have ethics committees, a local hospital committee member might be willing to serve this function. Alternatively, a local university or community college may have a qualified person to call upon to lead this initial ethics committee meeting.

Guidelines for Case Review

Before undertaking any case review, the committee should agree on some overall guidelines. Who may bring issues to the committee? How do people contact the committee? Will notes be kept? Will the committee simply operate as a forum for discussion, issue advisory opinions, or give directives for action? These guidelines should be made available to all staff members and may be formalized in a document identifying ethics committee procedures. Ongoing case review may be conducted as needed by a small group of committee members and reported to the whole committee at its next meeting. Alternatively, some committees conduct case review as a committee of the whole.

Generally, cases brought to the ethics committee will have the form of "What should I do?" Genuine quandaries often arise from new situations or situations not covered by professional training or left unclear in agency policies. Less often, cases of personnel conflict will come to the committee. Some agencies allow cases to be referred only by staff members; others might allow patients and families to use this resource. In all cases, it is advisable to have the chairperson review the case ahead of time and determine that the issue really does involve questions of ethics and values and is not something that would be better handled as a personnel matter, a communication problem, or an issue that falls under an existing agency policy.

If legal or regulatory issues are involved, professional organizations or a lawyer should be consulted before the case review is conducted. During the case discussion, it is important to be systematic: articulate a clear question to be answered, ascertain the facts of the case, hear different parties if it involves some kind of conflict, and elicit possible solutions with the pros and cons of each. The discussion should maintain confidentiality by using initials in place of full patient names. The chairperson should allow ample time for consideration of various viewpoints, concluding the discussion when a consensus emerges.

Two things are most important. The first is that the atmosphere be one of collaboration and respect, with all efforts made to avoid personal attacks and divisiveness, even when there is a serious difference of opinion. The second is that the discussion should focus on the reasons that can be given for and against a particular position. Reasons may have to do with patient, staff, or family rights or a calculation of costs and benefits [cf. Chapter 1]. Keeping the focus on reasons helps to diffuse an emotional situation, with the discussion centering on whether a reason is compelling rather than who presented the position. Moreover, understanding another person's reasons may increase respect for that person's views and may lead to a change of opinion on the part of the listeners, thus making consensus more likely.

One of the hallmarks of ethics discussions, which should be understood by all participants, is that there still may be irreconcilable differences of values even after extensive discussion. If the discussion seems to have gone as far as it can go with no clear consensus, there are several options to pursue. Individuals can just agree to disagree. But that will not answer the ethical question unless it is a situation where the nurse may have discretion to follow her own view. Another possible option is for participants to agree to go with the majority view, with the acknowledgment that if this requires an individual to act against conscience or against what she sees as professional obligation, she may remove herself from the case. A third possibility, especially if the issue is one that may be encountered again, is to have the agency develop a policy that outlines appropriate responses to the problem.

A Final Recommendation

To be successful in facilitating ethical caring for home health care patients, collaborative solutions to ethical quandaries, and conflict resolution, ethics committees must have sincere support from agency leadership. Sufficient resources should be dedicated to providing the materials, educational programs, and practical support that is essential to the operation of a home health care ethics committee.

GLOSSARY

Abandonment: The improper termination of the relationship between a professional caregiver and patient.

Advance directive: A legal document through which a competent individual may provide directions and wishes about medical care or name a proxy who has the authority to make medical decisions. It is used when the person is unable to make or communicate decisions about medical treatment and prepared before any condition or circumstance occurs that renders the patient incapable of actively making a decision regarding medical care.

Allow Natural Death Order: A physician's order that instructs healthcare professionals to withhold or withdraw life-sustaining technologies from a terminally ill patient and allow death to occur.

Assent: A weakened form of consent given by minors.

Assisted suicide: Assisting a patient by providing the means for the individual to take his or her own life.

Authenticity: In cases of substituted judgment, the concept of authenticity requires that decisions be made for patients that are consistent with their values and the way they lived their lives.

Autonomy: The right to determine what happens to one's own body based on one's values. Autonomous decisions are free, deliberate, informed, and lead to self-governed action.

Battery: The unlawful touching of another person without the individual's permission. Battery occurs in the context of medical care when the treatment exceeds what the patient has consented to, constituting technical battery for which the patient may seek redress.

Beneficence: Doing or promoting good and well-being.

Benevolent deception: Deceiving or withholding information in order to benefit the patient.

Best interest standard: A decision by a surrogate decision maker based on what would be in the patient's best interest.

Breach: Failure to meet a legal duty either by acting or failing to act.

Breach of Confidence: The legal term for a breach of confidentiality.

Closed awareness: The situation when a patient understands his or her condition or prognosis, but does not talk about it.

Code of ethics: Codes put forward by professional organizations, outlining responsibilities in the context of professional-patient relationships.

Collaborative decision-making: The process whereby patients retain their central role in making final decisions for themselves but reach their decisions after consultation with their families or others.

Comfort One: A program enacted to allow patients to signal treatment refusal by wearing bracelets in cases where the individual becomes incapacitated and is unable to communicate end-of-life wishes.

Community Mental Health Centers Act: Legislation enacted in 1963 which established the goal of transferring patients out of psychiatric institutions to live in the community.

Competence: The mental ability to make judgments based on a certain level of rationality; decisional capacity.

Compliance: A patient or family's adherence with a plan of care prescribed by professional caregivers.

Compromise decision-making: A decision-making process in which competent patients who have clear ideas about what they want are willing to shape their decisions in response to the wishes of others through a process of negotiation and compromise.

Confidentiality: Informational privacy between health care professionals and their patients.

Consequentialist ethical theories: Ethical theories which maintain that the rightness and wrongness of actions is determined solely by their consequences. Acts are considered right if they produce better consequences for everyone involved than any alternative act.

Conservator of the person: Someone appointed by the Probate Court when the Court finds that a person is incapable of making decisions about his or her healthcare. This person has the power to give consent for medical care, treatment, and services provided to the incapable person.

Cultural competence: The ability to provide culturally sensitive and appropriate care, based on knowledge of cultural views and values and appreciation for cultural differences.

Damages: Monetary compensation awarded by the courts for injury sustained to one's body or property due to negligence on the part of another party who owed a duty.

Death with Dignity Act: Oregon legislation which legalizes physician-assisted suicide.

DNR Code: Indicates "do not resuscitate" in the event of cardiac arrest. Also referred to as "no code."

Doctrine of double effect: The Christian doctrine according to which acts having both good and bad consequences are morally permissible, even if the bad consequences are known beforehand, as long as the intention is to bring about good. Such acts must be good or morally neutral in and of themselves. The bad consequences cannot be used as a means to bring about the good, and the good consequences must be proportionate to or greater than the bad consequences.

Dual diagnosis patient: A psychiatric patient who has been diagnosed with both a mental health condition and a substance abuse problem.

Durable Power of Attorney for Health Care: A type of advance directive in which a person is designated as a patient's decision-maker for medical questions that arise if the patient becomes incapacitated.

Emancipated minor: Someone under the age of majority who lives independently of his or her parents. An emancipated minor can legally consent to treatment and is responsible for his or her own debts.

Ethical Dilemma: An ethical problem that results from conflicting moral ideals.

Ethical Relativism: The view that there are no culturally independent moral truths. What is right or wrong depends on or varies with the time, place, or cultural group.

Ethics Committee: An advisory or consultative committee that provides a forum for discussing ethical issues and offers advice on appropriate actions. Ethics committees have been established by hospitals and home health care agencies.

Ethics of care: An ethical theory that identifies caring as the essential moral guideline. This theory focuses on the value of caring, emotional response and sensitivity, values caring relationships, and attends to the particulars of situations rather than relying on the application of traditional moral principles.

Euthanasia: The intentional taking of another's life or the refraining from acts that could prolong another's life out of considerations of mercy. Active euthanasia involves an action intended to hasten death in order to relieve suffering, whereas allowing death to occur by withholding or withdrawing treatment that could prolong a person's life is passive euthanasia.

Extraordinary means: Means used to prolong a patient's life where the physical, emotional, and financial burdens outweigh the benefits of the treatment.

Futile treatment: Treatment that will not provide any medical benefit.

Gravely disabled: An individual who is unable to provide food, shelter, and clothing for himself or herself due to mental illness.

Guardian *ad litem*: A guardian appointed on behalf of someone who is incapacitated.

Health care agent: A person authorized in a Durable Power of Attorney for Health Care directive to make medical decisions on behalf of the patient when the patient has become incapacitated.

Heroic measures: Extraordinary means used to prolong a person's life.

HIPAA: Health Insurance Portability and Accountability Act of 1996; federal legislation which, in addition to other provisions, requires protection for private medical information.

Hospice: A program of end-of-life care focused on relief of symptoms and suffering.

Implicit/implied consent: Non-verbal consent to treatment, e.g., by physical cooperation.

Individualistic decision-making: Decision-making process where patients think through the issues independently and reach a unilateral decision.

Informed consent: A competent patient's permission to provide medical care following disclosure of relevant information, requiring the capacity on the part of the patient to make a decision, an understanding of the information presented, and the absence of coercion.

Incompetence: The physical or mental incapacity to carry out one's affairs. Incompetent patients cannot enter into contracts. Strictly speaking, incompetence must be determined by a court.

***In loco parentis*:** In the place of a parent, instead of a parent, charged with parents' rights, duties, and responsibilities.

JCAHO: Joint Commission on Accreditation of Healthcare Organizations. The body charged with accrediting hospitals and other health care agencies

Least restrictive alternative: The treatment setting that provides the fewest limits on physical freedom and activities.

Legalism: The view that right and wrong are fully determined by the legal requirements that apply to a situation.

Life support system: A form of treatment that delays the time of death or maintains the patient in a state of permanent unconsciousness. These include among others: respirators and dialysis, cardiopulmonary resuscitation, artificial nutrition and hydration, and antibiotics in certain circumstances.

Living Will: A legal document that states whether a person wishes to have administered life-sustaining procedures or treatments in the event of a terminal condition. A Living Will goes into effect only when (1) the individual is unable to make or communicate decisions about health care and (2) is in a terminal condition.

Mandatory Treatment: Treatment ordered by a court when a patient is dangerous to self or others.

Malpractice: Professional misconduct or unreasonable lack of skills

Mature Minor Doctrine: Legal status given under common law for minors to consent to care.

Medical Community Model: A standard of disclosure which requires physicians to disclose only those risks that are consistent with the practice of the local community.

Moral Distress: The anguish nurses experience when they feel they are prevented from acting according to their judgments about what it is morally right to do.

Negligence: A failure to use reasonable care.

Nonadherence: Noncompliance with a plan of care.

Palliative Care: Care aimed at relieving pain and suffering.

***Parens patriae*:** The principle that the state must care for those who cannot care for themselves.

Paternalism: The infringement of a patient's autonomy for his or her own good. Also referred to as "parentalism."

Permanently unconscious: The condition of being in a permanent coma or persistent vegetative state where the patient is unaware of himself or herself or the surroundings and is unresponsive.

***Prima facie* rights:** At first sight; these rights are capable of being overridden by more stringent rights.

Privacy: The right to live without unwarranted interference by the public; the right to be left alone.

PSDA: Patient Self-Determination Act. Federal legislation that recognizes patients' rights to refuse medical treatment, even if death would result, and requires health care facilities to maintain policies and procedures consistent with advance directives.

Reasonable Person Standard: The standard used in judging for incompetent individuals based on what a reasonable, prudent person would do under the circumstances.

Right: A claim against others.

Rights-based ethical theories: Ethical theories that define right acts as those that conform to the moral and legal rights of individuals.

Shared decision making: A decision-making process in which patients share the task of deciding what to do with families and others. This process may involve compromise or collaboration.

Self-determination: The capacity and right to make decisions for oneself.

Standard of care: Requires acting as a reasonable, prudent nurse would act in similar circumstances.

Substituted judgment standard: The standard according to which a surrogate decision-maker acts on the basis of what the patient would have done if competent.

Suicide: The intentional taking of one's own life.

Supererogatory: Above and beyond the call of duty. Supererogatory acts are both praiseworthy and nonobligatory.

Surrogate decision-maker: The proxy or substitute decision maker for the patient.

Terminal condition: A condition (1) that is incurable and irreversible and (2) that will result in death in a relatively short time if life support systems are not provided.

Therapeutic privilege: Withholding medical information, based on the contention that disclosure would complicate or hinder treatment, pose psychological damage to the patient, or render the patient incapable of rational decision making.

Tort: A private or civil wrong or injury, including breach of contract.

Tort liability: Professional liability resulting from a duty toward the patient, a breach of duty, and the breach causing the patient's injuries.

Waiver of a right: Relinquishing a right.

BIBLIOGRAPHY

Books

Andrews, Margaret M. and Boyle, Joyceen S. (Eds.): *Transcultural Concepts in Nursing Care*, 3rd ed. Philadelphia: J. B. Lippencott Company, 1999.

Arras, John D., Porterfield, H. William, and Porterfield, Linda Obenauf (Eds.): *Bringing the Hospital Home: Ethical and Social Implications of High-Tech Home Care*. Baltimore and London: Johns Hopkins University, 1995.

Beauchamp, Tom L., and Childress, James F.: *Principles of Biomedical Ethics*, 5th ed. New York: Oxford University Press, 2001.

Benjamin, Martin, and Curtis, Joy: *Ethics in Nursing*, 3rd ed. New York: Oxford University, 1992.

Benner, Patricia: *From Novice to Expert: Excellence and Power in Clinical Nursing Practice*. Menlo Park, CA.: Addison-Wesley, 1984.

_____and Wrubel, J.: *The Primacy of Caring: Stress and Coping in Health and Illness*. Menlo Park, CA: Addison-Wesley, 1989.

Bishop, Anne H., and Scudder, Jr., John R. (Eds.): *Caring, Curing, Coping: Nurse, Physician, Patient, Relationship*. Birmingham, AL: University of Alabama, 1985.

_____: *Nursing Ethics: Holistic Caring Practice*, 2nd ed. Boston: Jones and Bartlett, 2001.

Clemen-Stone, Susan, McGuire, Sandra L., and Eigsti, Diane Gerber (Eds.): *Comprehensive Community Health Nursing. Family, Aggregate, and Community Practice*, 6th ed. St. Louis, MO: Mosby, 2002.

Davis, Anne J., Aroskar, Mila A., Liaschenko, Joan, and Drought, Theresa S., (Eds.): *Ethical Dilemmas and Nursing Practice*, 4th ed. Upper Saddle River, NJ: Prentice-Hall, 1997.

Galanti, Geri-Ann: *Caring for Patients from Different Cultures: Case Studies from American Hospitals*, 3rd ed. Philadelphia: University of Pennsylvania, 2003.

Giger, J., and Davidhizar, R. (Eds.) *Transcultural Nursing: Assessment and Intervention*, 4th ed. New York: Mosby, 2003.

Gubrium, Jaber F., and Sankar, K. Pal: *The Home Care Experience*. Thousand Oaks, CA: Sage, 1990.

Haddad, Amy Marie, and Kapp, Marshall B.: *Ethical and Legal Issues in Home Care: Case Studies and Analyses*. Norwalk, CT: Appleton and Lange, 1991.

Hammond, John S., Keeney, Ralph L., and Raiffa, Howard: *Smart Choices: A Practical Guide to Making Better Decisions*. Boston: Harvard Business School Press, 1999.

Henderson, Virginia: *The Nature of Nursing.* New York: MacMillan, 1991.

Jameton, Andrew: *Nursing Practice: The Ethical Issues,* Englewood Cliffs, NJ: Prentice-Hall, 1984.

Kane, Rosalie A., and Caplan, Arthur L: *Everyday Ethics: Resolving Dilemmas in Nursing Home Life.* New York: Springer, 1990.

Keltner, Norman L., Schwecke, Lee Hilyard, and Bostrom, Carol E.: *Psychiatric Nursing,* 4th ed. St. Louis, MO: Mosby, 2006.

Leininger, M. M., and McFarland, M. R.: *Transcultural Nursing: Concepts, Theories, Research and Practice,* 3rd ed. New York: McGraw-Hill, Medical Pub. Division, 2002.

Marrelli, Tina M.: *Hospice and Palliative Care Handbook. Quality, Compliance, and Reimbursement,* 2nd ed. St. Louis, MO: Mosby, 2004.

Moody, Harry R.: *Ethics in an Aging Society.* Baltimore: John Hopkins University, 1996.

Nelson, James Lindemann, and Nelson, Hilde Lindemann: *The Patient in the Family: An Ethics of Medicine and Families.* New York: Routledge, 1995.

Parks, Jennifer A.: *No Place Like Home: Feminist Ethics and Home Health Care,* Bloomington, IN: Indiana University Press, 2003.

Potter, Patricia A., and Perry, Anne Griffin.: *Fundamentals of Nursing,* 6th ed. St. Louis, MO: Mosby, 2006.

Rice, Robin. *Home Health Nursing Practice Concepts and Application,* 4th ed. St. Louis, MO: Mosby, 2006.

Robbins, Dennis A.: *Ethical and Legal Issues in Home Health and Long Term Care: Challenges and Solutions,* Gaithersburg, MD: Aspen, 1996.

Russo, J. Edward, and Schoemaker, Paul J. H.: *Decision Traps: The Ten Barriers to Brilliant Decision-Making and How to Overcome Them.* New York: a Fireside edition, Simon and Schuster, 1989.

Stanhope, Marcia, and Lancaster, Jeannette: *Foundations of Nursing in the Community,* 2nd ed. Wilmette: Mosby, 2006.

Swanson, Janice M., and Albrecht, Mary. *Community Health Nursing: Promoting the Health of Aggregates.* Philadelphia: W.B. Saunders, 1993.

Tong, Rosemarie: *Feminist Thought: A More Comprehensive Introduction,* Boulder, CO: Westview Press, 1998.

Watson, Jean: *Nursing: the Philosophy and Science of Caring,* Boston: Little, Brown, 1979.
_____: *Nursing: Human Science and Human Care: A Theory of Nursing,* Norwalk, CT: Appleton-Century-Crofts, 1985.

White, Gladys B., (Ed.): *Ethical Dilemmas in Contemporary Nursing Practice.* Washington, DC: American Nurses, 1992.

Wilson, Holly Skodol, and Kneisl, Carol Ren: *Psychiatric Nursing,* 5th ed., Menlo Park, CA: Addison-Wesley Nursing, a division of the Benjamin Cummings Publishing Company, 1996.

Wong, Donna L., Hockenberry-Eaton, Marilyn, Wilson, David, Winkelstein, Marilyn L., and Schwartz, Patricia: *Wong's Essentials of Pediatric Nursing,* 7th Edition. St Louis, MO: Mosby, 2005.

Articles and Chapters

American Academy of Pediatrics: Guidelines for home care. *Pediatrics, 74*:434–436, 1995.

Benner, Patricia, and Gordon, Suzanne: Caring practice. *Caregiving: Readings in Knowledge, Practice, Ethics, and Politics,* ed. Gordon, Suzanne, Benner, Patricia, and Noddings, Nel. Philadelphia: University of Pennsylvania Press, 1996.

Betancourt, J., Green, A., and Carrillo, J.: Cultural competence in health care: Emerging frameworks and practical approaches. Field Report, The Commonwealth Fund, 2002.

Callahan, Joan: Families as care-givers: limits of morality in care-giving. In Jecker, Nancy (Ed.): *Aging and Ethics: Philosophical Problems in Gerontology.* Totowa, Humana, 1992.

Cameron, Miriam E.: Value, be, do: Guidelines for resolving ethical conflict. *Journal of Nursing Law, 6* (4), 15-24, 2000.

Collopy, Bart, Dubler, Nancy, and Zuckerman, Connie: The ethics of home care: Autonomy and accommodation. *Hastings Center Report,* March/April 1990.

Corley, Mary C.: Nurse moral distress: A proposed theory and research agenda. *Nursing Ethics, 9* (6), 2002.

_____, Elswick, R.K., Gorman, Martha, and Clor, Theresa. Development and evaluation of a moral distress scale. *Journal of Advanced Nursing, 33* (2), 250–256, 2001.

Erlen, J.A.: Ethics. Moral distress; A pervasive problem. *Orthopedic Nursing, 20* (2), 76-80, 2001.

Flowers, Deborah L.: Culturally competent nursing care. A challenge for the 21st century. *Critical Care Nurse, 24* (4), August 2004.

Fry, Sara T.: The role of caring in a theory of nursing ethics. In Holmes, Helen Bequaert; and Purdy, Laura M. (Eds.): *Feminist Perspectives in Medical Ethics.* Bloomington and Indianapolis, Indiana University Press, 1992.

Green-Hernandez, Carol, Quinn, Agatha A., Denman-Vitale, Susan, Falkenstern, Sharon K., and Judge-Ellis, Tess: Making primary care culturally competent. *The Nurse Practitioner, 29* (6), 49–55, 2004.

Hanna, D.R. Moral Distress: The state of the science. *Nurse Manager, 18* (1), 73–93, 2004.

Jameton, Andrew: Dilemmas of moral distress: Moral responsibility; and nursing practice. *AWHONN's Clinical Issues in Perinatal and Women's Health Nursing, 4* (4), 542–551, 1993.

Jecker, Nancy: Role of intimate others. In Jecker *op. cit.*

Ladd Rosalind Ekman, Pasquerella, Lynn, and Smith, Sheri: What to do when the end is near: Ethical issues in home health care nursing. *Public Health Nursing, 17* (2): 103–110, 2000.

Lantos, John, and Kohrman, Arthur F.: Ethical aspects of pediatric home care. *Pediatrics, 89*:920–24, 1992.

Leonard, Barbara J., and Plotnikoff, Gregory A.: Awareness: The heart of cultural competence. A*ACN Clinical Issues, 11* (1), pp. 51–59, 2000.

Mazanec, Polly, and Tyler, Mary Kay: cultural considerations in end-of-life care. *American Journal of Nursing, 103* (30): 50–58, 2003.

Nathaniel, A.: Moral distress among nurses. *The American Nurses Association Ethics & Human Rights Issues Update* Retrieved from http://www.nursingworld.org/ethics/update/vol1no3a.htm, 2002.

Okun, Ale: All in the family: the inequity between parental rights and home care duties. In Cassidy, Robert (Ed.): *Pediatric Ethics: From Principles to Practice.* Amsterdam: Harwood, 1996.

Rew, L., Becker, H., Cookston, J., Khosropour, S., and Martinex, S.: Measuring cultural awareness in nursing students. *Journal of Nursing Education, 42* (6), 2003.

Salimbene, Suzanne: Cultural Competence: A priority for performance Improvement Action. *Journal of Nursing Care Quality, 13* (3), 23–25, 1999.

Stulginsky, M.M.: Nurses home health experience. *Nursing and Health Care, 14*:405, 1993.

Watson, Jean: New dimensions of human caring theory. *Nursing Science Quarterly, 1*: 175, 1988.

Wilkinson, J.M.: Moral distress in nursing practice: Experience and effect. *Nursing Forum, 23* (1), 16-29, 1987/88.

Professional Codes, State Regulations, and Legal Cases

American Nurses Association, *Code of Ethics for Nurses with Interpretive Statements*, Washington, D.C., ANA Publications, 2001.

_____.: *Bill of Rights for Registered Nurses*, 2001.

_____.: *Nursing and the Patient Self-Determination Act*, 1991.

_____.: *Nursing's Social Policy Statement*, Second Edition.

_____.: *On Nursing Care and Do-Not-Resuscitate Decisions*, 2003.

_____.: *Privacy and Confidentiality*, 2006.

Cruzan v. Director, Missouri Dept. of Health, 110 S. Ct. 2841, 1990.

Foy v. Greenblott, 141 Cal. App. 3d 1, 13, 1983.

International Council of Nurses, *Code of Ethics for Nurses*, Geneva, Switzerland, 2006.

Jaffe v. Redmond, 518 S. Ct. 1, 1996.

Lampe v. Presbyterian Medical Center, 41 Colo. App. 465 P2d 513, 1978.

State of Rhode Island and Providence Plantations. Department of Health. *Rules and Regulations for the Licensing of Professional Registered, Certified Registered Nurse Practitioners, Certified Registered Nurse Anesthetists, and Practical Nurses and Standards for the Approval of Basic Nursing Education Programs*, 2004.

Tarasoff v. Board of Regents of University of California, 529 P 2d 553 CA, 1976.

Tuma v. Board of Nursing, 100 Idaho 74, 593 P. 2d. 711, 1979.

Warthen v. Toms River Community Memorial Hospital, 101 N.J. 255, 501 A.2d 926 N.J., 1985.

Oregon Nurses Association, *Position Paper on the Death with Dignity Act*, 1995. Retrieved from oregonrn.org.

Media Resources

Cultural Competence, Irvine, CA: Concept Media, 2006.

Web Sites

http://nursingworld.org/ethics/
http://www.cybernurse.com/books/nursingethics.html

INDEX

ABOUT THE AUTHORS

Rosalind Ekman Ladd is Emerita Professor of Philosophy, Wheaton College, Norton, Massachusetts, and Lecturer in Pediatrics, the Warren Alpert Medical School, Brown University. She is co-author of *Ethical Dilemmas in Pediatrics: A Case Study Approach* and editor of *Children's Rights Re-visioned: Philosophical Readings.* She has published on medical ethics, children's rights, and women's rights in health care. She serves on Ethics Committees of three hospitals in Rhode Island and has wide experience as lecturer, workshop leader, and consultant.

Lynn Pasquerella is Provost at the University of Hartford. She is a graduate of Mount Holyoke College (A.B.) and Brown University (Ph.D.). Professor Pasquerella is was chosen by the American Association of Higher Education and *Change* Magazine as one of the "Young Leaders of the Academy." She serves on the Institutional Review Board of the Rhode Island State Health Department and on the Ethics Committee of Day Kimball Hospital. She has published extensively in the areas of theoretical and applied ethics, public policy, medical ethics, and the philosophy of law. Her current research focuses on the ethical and legal issues related to biobanking.

Sheri Smith received her B.A. in Biology and Philosophy from Millikin University and an A.M. and Ph.D. in Philosophy from Brown University. She is a Professor of Philosophy at Rhode Island College. Professor Smith has served on the Rhode Island Department of Health's Institutional Review Board, Genetic Screening Advisory Committee, and Allocation of Scarce Resources Pandemic Flu Committee. She is a member of the Board of Trustees of Roger Williams Hospital and has served on the Institutional Review Board and as chair of the Ethics Advisory Committee of Roger Williams Medical Center. She has published numerous articles in the area of bioethics. She is a specialist in the field of nursing ethics and has presented several workshops for nurses working in hospitals, home health care agencies, and hospices. Professor Smith has also contributed as an essayist and commentator for Trinity Repertory Company's Humanities Series.

In addition to their individual work, the authors have collaborated on several articles and papers that were presented at national and international conferences:

"Infants, the Dead Donor Rule, and Organ Donation: Should the Rules Be Changed?" in *Law, Medicine and Ethics*, Volume 20, Number 3, (September 2001) and in *Proceedings of the Thirteenth World Congress on Medical Law*, Helsinki, Finland (August 2000). Pages 888-892.

"What to Do When the End is Near: Ethical Issues in Home Health Care" in *Public Health Nursing*, Volume 17, Number 2, (2000). Pages 103-110.

"In the Interest of the Fetus: Mandatory Prenatal Classes in the Workplace" in *Women and Politics*, Volume 13, Number 3/4, (1993). Pages 191-201. Reprinted in Janna Merrick, ed., *The Politics of Pregnancy: Issues in the Maternal-Fetal Relationship.* Haworth Press, 1994. Pages 191-201.

"Liability-Driven Ethics: The Impact on Hiring Practices" in *Business Ethics Quarterly*, Volume 4, Issue 3, (1994). Pages 321-333.

Charles C Thomas
PUBLISHER • LTD.

P.O. Box 19265
Springfield, IL 62794-9265

Book Savings* Save 10%, Save 15%, Save 20%!

- Geldard, Kathryn & David Geldard—**PERSONAL COUNSELING SKILLS: An Integrative Approach.** '08, 282 pp. (7 x 10), 20 il., 3 tables, paper.

- Kendler, Howard H.—**AMORAL THOUGHTS ABOUT MORALITY: The Intersection of Science, Psychology, and Ethics. (2nd Ed.)** '08, 246 pp. (7 x 10).

- Plach, Tom—**INVESTIGATING ALLEGATIONS OF CHILD AND ADOLESCENT SEXUAL ABUSE: An Overview for Professionals.** '08, 172 pp. (7 x 10).

- Bryan, Willie V.—**MULTICULTURAL ASPECTS OF DISABILITIES: A Guide to Understanding and Assisting Minorities in the Rehabilitation Process. (2nd Ed.)** '07, 348 pp. (7 x 10). $69.95, hard, $49.95, paper.

- Crandell, John M. Jr. & Lee W. Robinson—**LIVING WITH LOW VISION AND BLINDNESS: Guidelines That Help Professionals and Individuals Understand Vision Impairments.** '07, 220 pp. (7 x 10), 14 il., $49.95, hard, $34.95, paper.

- Daniels, Thomas & Allen Ivey—**MICROCOUNSELING: Making Skills Training Work In a Multicultural World.** '07, 296 pp. (7 x 10), 12 il., 3 tables, $65.95, hard, $45.95, paper.

- France, Kenneth—**CRISIS INTERVENTION: A Handbook of Immediate Person-to-Person Help. (5th Ed.)** '07, 320 pp. (7 x 10), 3 il., $65.95, hard, $45.95, paper.

- Malouff, John M. & Nicola S. Schutte—**ACTIVITIES TO ENHANCE SOCIAL, EMOTIONAL, AND PROBLEM-SOLVING SKILLS: Seventy-six Activities That Teach Children, Adolescents, and Adults Skills Crucial to Success in Life. (2nd Ed.)** '07, 248 pp. (8 1/2 x 11), 3 il., $44.95, spiral (paper).

- Gardner, Richard A., S. Richard Sauber & Demosthenes Lorandos—**THE INTERNATIONAL HANDBOOK OF PARENTAL ALIENATION SYNDROME: Conceptual, Clinical and Legal Considerations.** '06, 476 pp. (8 1/2 x 11), 12 il., 10 tables, $84.95, hard.

- Henderson, George; Dorscine Spigner-Littles & Virginia Hall Milhouse—**A PRACTITIONER'S GUIDE TO UNDERSTANDING INDIGENOUS AND FOREIGN CULTURES: An Analysis of Relationships Between Ethnicity, Social Class and Therapeutic Intervention Strategies. (3rd Ed.)** '06, 352 pp. (7 x 10), 1 il., 1 table, $66.95, hard, $46.95, paper.

- Paton, Douglas & David Johnston—**DISASTER RESILIENCE: An Integrated Approach.** '06, 344 pp. (7 x 10), 22 il., 9 tables, $68.95, hard, $48.95, paper.

- Phillips, Norma Kolko & Shulasmith Lala Ashenberg Straussner—**CHILDREN IN THE URBAN ENVIRONMENT: Linking Social Policy and Clinical Practice. (2nd Ed.)** '06, 300 pp. (7 x 10), 2 tables, $67.95, hard, $47.95, paper.

- Roberts, Albert R. & David W. Springer—**SOCIAL WORK IN JUVENILE AND CRIMINAL JUSTICE SETTINGS. (3rd Ed.)** '06, 462 pp. (8 x 10), 7 il., (1 in color), 17 tables, $69.95, paper.

- Soby, Jeanette M.—**PRENATAL EXPOSURE TO DRUGS/ALCOHOL: Characteristics and Educational Implications of Fetal Alcohol Syndrome and Cocaine/Polydrug Effects. (2nd Ed.)** '06, 188 pp. (7 x 10), 7 il., 21 tables, $44.95, hard, $28.95, paper.

- Mayers, Raymond Sanchez—**FINANCIAL MANAGEMENT FOR NONPROFIT HUMAN SERVICE ORGANIZATIONS. (2nd Ed.)** '04, 354 pp. (7 x 10), 19 il., 46 tables, $75.95, hard, $55.95, paper.

- Curtis, Judith A.—**THE RENAL PATIENT'S GUIDE TO GOOD EATING: A Cookbook for Patients by a Patient. (2nd Ed.)** '03, 226 pp. (7 x 10), 30 il., $36.95, (spiral) paper.

- Richard, Michael A. & William G. Emener—**I'M A PEOPLE PERSON: A Guide to Human Service Professions.** '03, 262 pp. (8 x 10), 2 il., 5 tables, $57.95, hard, $38.95, paper.

- Ladd, Rosalind Ekman, Lynn Pasquerella, and Sheri Smith—**ETHICAL ISSUES IN HOME HEALTH CARE.** '02, 208 pp. (7 x 10), $48.95, hard, $31.95, paper.

- Thompson, Richard H.—**PSYCHOSOCIAL RESEARCH ON PEDIATRIC HOSPITALIZATION AND HEALTH CARE: A Review of the Literature.** '85, 364 pp., 1 il., $43.95, paper.

- Thompson, Richard H. & Gene Stanford—**CHILD LIFE IN HOSPITALS: Theory and Practice.** '81, 284 pp., 1 table, $41.95, paper.

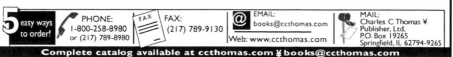

5 easy ways to order!

PHONE: 1-800-258-8980 or (217) 789-8980

FAX: (217) 789-9130

EMAIL: books@ccthomas.com
Web: www.ccthomas.com

MAIL: Charles C Thomas ¥ Publisher, Ltd. P.O. Box 19265 Springfield, IL 62794-9265

Complete catalog available at ccthomas.com ¥ books@ccthomas.com

Books sent on approval ¥ Shipping charges: $7.75 min. U.S. / Outside U.S., actual shipping fees will be charged ¥ Prices subject to change without notice

*Savings include all titles shown here and on our web site. For a limited time only.